Fruit Infused Water

Easy Vitamin Water Recipes for Weight Loss

(Detox and Metabolism Boosting Vitamin Water)

Eddy Houston

I0136065

Published By **Simon Dough**

Eddy Houston

Fruit Infused Water: Easy Vitamin Water Recipes for Weight Loss (Detox and Metabolism Boosting Vitamin Water)

ISBN   978-1-7388267-7-3

No part of this guidebook shall be reproduced in any form without permission in writing from the publisher except in the case of brief quotations embodied in critical articles or reviews.

Legal & Disclaimer

Table Of Contents

Chapter 1: Why Do People Drink Fruit Infused

Water?

Before I answer this query, I am going to tell you what fruit infused water is.

What is fruit infused water?

When you had entered a spa for the very first time, have been you supplied with a tiny glass of water, which while sipped tasted like fruit? That is the fruit infused water that this ebook will let you know all approximately! At the forestall of the ebook, you may be for the motive that this fruit infused water is a tall glass that allows in smooth and nourishing you. The best detail approximately ingesting fruit infused water is that you could make it at home!

When you've got come lower back from a tough day at paintings or have completed your chores for the day, you're longing for a few element to appease your thirst. You will reach out to a glass of water, but skip it at times as it does not provide any flavor. This is whilst you may use fruit infused water due to the fact you will be able to revitalize your body. You recognise that there is no drink on the face of the planet which can update water. Mix that up with the vitamins and minerals that the culmination offer you at the same time as fed on, and you've got got the amazing aggregate ever – fruit infused water! This water is a adorable aggregate that has all of the elements that you could want. The superb element about fruit infused water is that you may add any herbs to offer you that burst of taste! This is healthful and is the most inexpensive drink you could ever come across. You will have a look at the only of a type blessings that you may reap via ingesting fruit infused water. Let us now recognize why it's far super which you drink fruit infused water.

Why is fruit infused water the extraordinary drink?

The purpose we must drink water is to live hydrates. Another advantage of drinking water is that we can keep away from ingesting more meals. However, many a time human beings discover that water is bland to flavor and they may lose interest of it. Sometimes humans honestly do not experience consuming undeniable water due to the flavor. Hence, people lodge to caffeinated liquids or aerated drinks that have destructive results on someone. However, we can quench our thirst without resorting to either those drinks or water. The healthiest and one of the tastiest solutions to this trouble is fruit infused or herb infused water. They are clean to prepare and are also quite healthful. It is not always candy but is extremely sparkling. These drinks are flavorful and are powerful in quenching thirst.

In essence, the manner of infusing water is surely crushing herbs or cease end result and mixing them with water to fuse the flavors. It is without a doubt a more fit replacement to water than aerated drinks which have excessive amounts of sugar. Another advantage is that you may pick out out the flavor which you would like and infuse the water consequently.

Many people receive as real with that eating 8 glasses of water a day allows with weight reduction. However, it isn't clean to have 8 glasses an afternoon. So, you can drink infused water as an alternative. It has the identical impact with weight reduction. Also, because you could probably infuse the water with flavors you are keen on, consuming eight glasses of it will now not be that difficult.

How should you begin with this?

The technique of infusing water is pretty easy. In concept, it's miles possible to infuse any flavor into the water. There are many recipes that you may observe. These recipes will contain system like infusion bottles and pitchers, blenders. They encompass a large choice of elements as nicely. Most human beings pick out to preserve the manner as easy as viable. Since it is simply an opportunity to water, it's miles simply useful to preserve the preparation manner easy. Think approximately any not unusual fruit or vegetable that you like and infuse it. You can also add herbs and spices to the water. You can actually do not forget any combination and infuse water.

The simplest of recipes to infuse water contain only a few additives and take about a minute or . You will have to pick an infusion jar or pitcher, which is basically the box wherein you will make your infused water.

The greater modern infuser bottles had been designed to make the machine of infusion easy. However, they could show to be slightly at the steeply-priced aspect. Only purchase them if you need to devour infused water on a each day basis. Otherwise, a everyday area, which you could find out at domestic, will artwork simply great. The first-class problem is that the technique might get a touch grimy and you could must smooth up after. You can use quite a few device to mash the herbs, culmination and veggies. A mortar and pestle or a muddler will do the trick.

The materials generally embody water; end result, vegetables, herbs and honestly not regularly they even encompass spices. The desire of the fruit, vegetable, herb and spice is virtually as a good deal as you. You can pick out them in line with your alternatives. However, it is not beneficial to use bananas because their texture is as a substitute organization and it can be tough to overwhelm them. The system turns into fairly messy. You need to make certain that the end result are gentle and ripe. This will make sure that the flavor of the infused water may be correct. The maximum not unusual prevent end end result used for infusion are citrus fruits and berries due to the fact they will be quite fresh. Many humans moreover use pineapples and watermelons due to their sweetness. When it involves vegetables cucumber is most normally used. Add ice on your recipe as nicely. Also embody an herb or spice to liven topics up.

Once you have got were given decided on your factors, you may sooner or later go with the float directly to creating the infused water. The way more or lots plenty less remains the identical. In case you are making a large amount of infused water, use a jug or pitcher. You can use an infuser bottle for smaller portions. Fill it up with water. Add the chopped end end result, veggies, herbs and spices that you have picked. Make high quality that they may be chopped into small quantities for less complicated infusion. Another approach that you can observe is to puree your elements. Pass this puree through a sieve to collect exceptional the liquid element. Dilute this with water to achieve your infused water.

You will need loads of staying electricity for this manner. You will need to allow the aggregate to sit down for round 8 or 9 hours just so the flavors can get infused nicely. The longer you permit it sit down down, the more flavorful the final product may be. Some substances infuse quicker whilst in contrast to others. Citrus end end result are believed to infuse the fastest. Herbs, as a substitute, can take pretty some hours. Berries additionally take a long time however additionally they launch pigments that coloration the water.

Place the infused water inside the refrigerator. When you are serving it, add some ice to enhance its clean effect.

Benefits of Fruit Infused water

Have you ever tasted fruit infused water in advance than? This beverage isn't best tasty and clean however it additionally has a number of health blessings. Squeeze the fruit a bit earlier than together with it to the infuser pitcher for steeping. This will decorate its nutritional price. There are hundreds of numerous recipes and each one has its very very own advantages.

Given underneath are some of the health blessings of fruit infused water:

You start consuming more nutrients

When you infuse water with culmination and different substances, all of the vitamins from them get infused as well. Hence, infused water no longer exceptional tastes higher but is likewise loaded with vitamins, nutrients, minerals and antioxidants. It is virtually a much healthier possibility to strength liquids, aerated drinks and caffeinated beverages.

You can growth your immunity

As you apprehend, unique end result assist in stopping special styles of diseases. Therefore, relying on the components that you use, infused water can assist in combating various sicknesses starting from cardiovascular illnesses to neural ailments. The additives of give up cease result help in regulating the pH degree of the body and this in turn reduces the risks of most cancers.

You might be capable of gradual the developing old manner

As cited in advance, fruit infused water includes antioxidants. They assist in slowing down the growing antique approach. Another gain is that the antioxidants boom the producing of collagen that improves pores and skin tremendous and makes it easy and silky. It permits you revel in more more youthful.

You can decorate your metabolism

Fruits have certain compounds in them that assist in speeding up metabolism, which in flip motives you to burn greater energy. One of the brilliant fruit infused beverages for this motive is lemon infused water. It promotes the dearth of weight.

You can be capable of rid the greater frame weight

When in evaluation to everyday water, fruit infused water is said to be greater filling and nutritious. It has lesser energy and sugar than easy beverages and caffeinated beverages. Some end result additionally have the effect of decreasing your urge for meals and therefore you do not overeat. Hence, thru ingesting fruit infused water you could have extra manage on your weight and you may also prevent snacking in amongst meals.

You also can have greater power than ever earlier than!

Since fruit infused drinks are so nutritious, they provide us with huge amounts of power. Hence, it's far very powerful for athletes, sportspersons and people who go to the fitness center frequently. In reality, human beings accept as true with that the ones drinks can replace sports sports drinks absolutely. In addition to being a more healthy possibility, those drinks taste manner better than sports activities beverages.

A new addition in your weight loss plan

Fruit infused drinks upload variety on your diet plan. You can offer you with any aggregate of give up result, greens, herbs and spices. Since you can continually test with the flavor, it in no way gets silly and livens up your each day food regimen.

Any super health benefits

Infused water permits the body with digestion and moreover enables with awesome troubles within the belly. As cited in advance, those drinks can also help with weight reduction. They energize you and depart you feeling refreshed. They additionally assist in cleansing the severa structures of the body and have a cooling effect to your belly.

By now you are aware about the severa health blessings of fruit infused liquids. In addition to the health benefits, they may be scrumptious. When you begin eating those beverages you'll need to use the fundamental recipes. Later on, whilst you are acquainted with the manner, you can rent extra complicated recipes for better taste.

Chapter 2: Benefits Of Water And Fruit

In the remaining financial disaster, you had amassed the records which you wanted about fruit infused water. You had been moreover encouraged about the distinct blessings which you may gain on ingesting the water. But, why is it that you are requested first-class to combine end result in water?

Benefits of water

Water is the wonderful a part of absolutely everyone's healthy eating plan as it has numerous blessings, which help you, easy your device up! This phase covers the advantages of water an awesome manner to assist in reinforcing your notion.

-    Water is the excellent way to flush out any pollution that you can have for your frame. It is because of this that you are asked to drink loads of water just so you'll be able to remove pollution which is probably soluble in water. You might be able to put off any minerals or vitamins that would have gathered within the incorrect regions of your frame.

-     You may additionally have observed that your body has started out to warmness up and your cheeks are warmth after you've got exercised. It is the same in relation to the adjustments in climate. This is while water works wonders. It lets in in regulating the temperature of your body. You will also be capable of pinnacle off all of the water you out of place through sweat.

-     It is proper a good way to drink water whilst you are looking at acquiring healthful pores and skin. You will locate that it actually works higher than another splendor that announces to smooth your face off the pimples or the spots and scars. You will find out that your pores and skin has executed a glow that it in no way had earlier than at the same time as you consume a variety of water.

-     Water works nicely in lubricating your muscles and joints and additionally reduces the friction a number of the joints. When you consume little or no water, you may locate that you have insufferable cramps.

-     You will find yourself tremendously lively for the purpose that water allows in developing a stability inside the fluids which can be found for your body. You will find yourself agile and alert whilst you are hydrated properly.

-     Water works wonders with reference to developing your metabolic costs. It lets in within the quick digestion of meals, which would probably ensure that you in no way be bothered through constipation.

- You will locate which you rarely get migraines and headaches which can had been due to dehydration.

- Water is an vital detail that is vital for you even as you are looking at dropping weight. When you're dehydrated, your frame has a decrease price of synthesis of proteins that make your frame store masses greater power that results in a advantage in your weight. This is regularly forced with hunger which makes you eat more when in fact all your body dreams is water.

- When you have got were given diarrhea or dysentery, you will lose hundreds of fluid that desires to be replenished. If you do not top off the water, you'll be most important yourself in the path of graver effects.

It is due to this that it's far proper for guys to drink close to 6 to eight glasses of water every day at the identical time as ladies need to drink no longer much less than five to 6 glasses every day. You do now not need to keep on with this size and might drink as lots water as possible. The following are a few hints that you could use as dreams!

-    Make certain that you drink a tumbler of water before every meal. This will ensure which you do no longer over consume for the reason that you'll be complete. You can also be able to make sure which you stay hydrated.

-    Make certain which you supply a bottle of water with you anyplace it is that you are going.

-    If you find your self feeling hungry, you may drink water to quench that starvation. You also can be capable of keep away from the more power that you can benefit.

-    Make wonderful that you have a jug this is complete of the fruit infused water in the fridge to make certain that you drink this whenever you discover it hard to make one glass of the fruit infused water in case you are in a hurry.

Benefits of Fruit

Fruits are an important detail of a diet plan and are very critical because of the fact they nourish your body and also provide it with vitamins which may be vital in your fitness and inside the maintenance of your body.

-    Certain quit result – bananas, peaches and prunes – assist in the preservation of the blood stress due to the reality that they're rich in potassium.

-     It is crucial that you consume give up end end result which might be wealthy in fiber thinking about they help in decreasing any ldl ldl cholesterol for your blood and furthermore lessen the risk of buying coronary heart illnesses. These stop result assist in improving the feature of your bowels and moreover leave you with a sense of fullness that results inside the truth that you do not feel hungry that often.

-     The energy in culmination are very lots much less in massive variety or even if they will be present, they're wholesome and wanted through your body.

-     Folic acid in cease quit end result enables in improving the formation of the blood cells for your body. It is vital that pregnant girls eat those cease result. This additionally allows in lowering the opportunity of ailments much like the defects of neural tubes.

-     It is critical which you eat quit result with vitamin C in them thinking about the truth that they help within the boom of the tissues for your body thereby healing any wounds.

-     When you have got got were given masses of cease result to your food plan, you can discover that you have a discounted risk of buying diabetes and cardiovascular ailments.

- Fruits help in retaining your eyes wholesome and similarly they help in preventing any eye illnesses that can be associated with your age.

It is for those very motives that it's far important that you eat a weight loss plan that is wealthy in give up end result. There are some guidelines you may use as regards to consuming extra end result as a part of your healthy eating plan.

1. You will need to make certain which you purchase an great amount of stop end result at the same time as you go to the grocery store. You can constantly pick out to shop for frozen or canned surrender end result.

2. Make effective that you have a bowl of fruit positioned in your coffee and ingesting tables to make certain which you are endorsed to consume this shape of end end result.

three. Make certain which you break up a few fruit and leave it inside the refrigerator a great way to devour it later.

4. Make sure that you upload a few forestall result on your meals. You could upload quit stop result on your cereal or have a fruit proper earlier than you begin ingesting a meal. You can also have a fruit salad.

5. If you are hungry, you may eat fruit in region of eating any junk food.

6. Make certain which you devour dry cease stop result in case you cannot have smooth fruits. But, you have to make certain which you devour a amazing deal lesser of the dry quit result at the identical time as in comparison to the clean fruit.

Chapter 3: The Dos And Don'ts!

When you're decrease lower returned from paintings on an afternoon on the equal time as it is warmth, you could pick out out to devour a can of soda or carbonated beverages. It is right that the ones liquids do no longer some thing but purpose harm on your frame. The sodas which have claimed to be diet sodas are worse than the normal sodas and have to be avoided just like the plague. These sodas consist of a whole lot of artificial sweeteners that motive numerous illnesses.

When you consume a weight-reduction plan soda, you may discover that you haven't lost weight however have received weight as an alternative. You also can had been underneath the affect that you'll obtain a surge of electricity, this is proper, however it is also actual that you will be giving your body a dose of sugar that consequences in diabetes and coronary coronary heart ailments. It has been proven that your teeth additionally commonly tend to go to pot whilst you eat an excessive amount of of the soda. The soda reasons the tooth to lose their calcium content leaving them soft.

When you continue to drink the sodas, you can find out that your body has all started out out to crave more for the sodas leaving you in a cycle that is dangerous to you! When you buy any flavored water at the grocery store, you will discover that there are quite a few additives that have massive portions of sugar, which bring about diabetes. Flavored water is better than the sodas but they do no longer do tons assist either. You can consequently pick to be easy and hydrated through eating fruit infused water that you have made at domestic! You is probably very satisfied to apprehend that this water has no additives for the cause that you'll be making it your self! You is probably capable of detox your body as properly and is probably capable of rid your body of any pollutants!

You can also pick out out out to eat espresso each morning to wake yourself as a incredible deal as device yourself up for the day. You will no longer be harm an excessive amount of with the resource of the espresso but there may be the drug, caffeine, that is dangerous for you. Your frame may be harmed an excessive amount of thru manner of the drug. If you eat too much espresso you can discover your self nauseous and also will have heart palpitations. You will need to consequently, recall each sip of espresso you take. It is extraordinary to pick fruit infused water due to the fact you will be capable of hold your self smooth and satisfied.

How do you are making fruit infused water?

You may were experimenting with severa techniques to lose weight and to moreover live wholesome. But, this method is the first-class manner to shed kilos too! You can comply with the stairs given below while you are looking at making your very non-public fruit infused water.

Step 1

You will need to decide what form of fruit infused water you want and why you're choosing that unique type. Now, accumulate the culmination and location the give up bring about a jug complete of water and ice. Store it within the refrigerator. You will need to have a look at the positive regulations with reference to the equal:

- Use stop end result which may be ripe and glowing that allows you to advantage the remarkable flavor of the fruit.

- Make remarkable which you have nice herbs an terrific way to ensure that you could make the water an awful lot better.

- Make positive which you use jars at the same time as you are making the fruit infused water. Make certain that you have mason jars which have been embellished properly on the subject of serving visitors the water.

- You may also choose out to shop for first-rate fruit infusion bottles for the reason that that will help you supply the water all round with you.

- You need to apply a wood spoon so that it will aggregate the factors nicely collectively and to extract the juice from the fruit.

Step 2

You will need to characteristic cold water to the pitcher and ensure that the water that you have in the pitcher is the equal quantity that you want.

Step 3

You can upload what number of ever ice cubes you will need to.

Step 4

You want to slice the give up end result up into the size which you have determined on so that you can upload first-rate the preferred amount of fruit to the water. You do no longer want to make a pulpy drink and will want to ensure which you have the right amount of fruit.

Step 5

You will need to bruise the stop end result a piece a good way to make certain that the fruit has infused into the water.

Step 6

You will need to shake the pitcher with a view to supply the water a flavor. If you discover that the taste is the proper amount you can want to interrupt up greater fruit if you want to make certain that the flavor is in keeping with your flavor. If you locate which you want to function a touch sugar, keep away from that for the purpose that it's far first rate to function herbal syrups like maple syrup or honey. You will then need to depart it in the refrigerator for a few hours.

Step 7

You will want to pour the water into glasses and serve it with a hint garnish with some herbs. Now drink it up! You have your very non-public fruit infused water! You can try this with any fruit you will want while you don't forget that you may be capable of gather one-of-a-kind benefits. There are some that would improve your energy whilst there are others that paintings within the course of boosting your metabolism or your immunity by way of the use of the usage of flushing out the pollutants.

Chapter 4: Recipes For Fruit Infused Water

Apple infused Water recipes

Apple, Cucumber and Ginger Fusion Fruit Infusion water

This infused water infused with apple, cucumber and ginger is exceedingly effective in increasing your metabolism and it's miles consequently advocated to consume it if you have overeaten. It can also preserve you hydrated and increases your stamina. It also can assist with weight reduction.

Apples are pretty filling and so this drink will make sure you do not hold snacking on junk food and this enables in controlling your weight. The cucumbers assist in flushing out the pollutants in your body and preserve you hydrated. The ginger lets in in enhancing your metabolism and also will increase your power stages (stamina).

Ingredients

- 2 – three slices of apple

- 2 slices of cucumber

- Piece of chopped ginger

Instructions

- Place the additives in a bowl and mix them.

- Now area this mixture into an Aqua combination basket.

- Add water into the basket.

- Leave this mixture in the refrigerator for a while to get most refreshment.

Apple and Raspberry Fruit Infused Water

To have specific health, desirable digestion is an absolute have to. However, fighting digestive issues isn't easy. Apple and raspberry infused water is a drink that could help combat those problems regardless of the fact that. The raspberries have greater fiber than maximum fruits and function low sugar content material fabric material. They also have just a few power. Hence, they'll be suitable for people with diabetes and additionally for folks that are in search of to shed pounds. The apples then again have pectin, which permits in detoxifying the frame and moreover aids in digestion.

Ingredients

- 3 barely squeezed raspberries

- 3 thin slices of apple

Instructions

- Take an Aqua mixture basket. Place the apples and raspberries in it.

- Fill it up with water and mix it a bit bit.

- Let the aggregate stand for at the least an hour for infusion to take vicinity.

- If you infuse it in a unmarried day, it'll beautify the flavor of the drink.

- Once all the drink has been ate up, you can eat the fruit that has been left in the back of.

Apple and Cinnamon Spa Water Fruit infused Water

This drink lets in in developing the power stages of someone. It additionally permits in growing stamina. This drink is extraordinarily tasty and regulates the blood sugar stage as nicely. Here is the recipe to make apple and cinnamon spa water infused water. This drink is the pleasant for the reason that apple used consists of numerous antioxidants like Vitamin C and cinnamon consists of the assets wherein it can modify the blood sugar stages thereby preventing diabetes. You additionally may be capable of lessen the pain this is induced due to arthritis. When you decide, you will find out your self lots greater inexperienced and focused.

Ingredients

- four thinly sliced Apple (halved)

- ½ Cinnamon stick

Instructions

- Take a container and blend the materials collectively.

- Now take this aggregate and area it in an Acquablend bottle.

- Fill the complete bottle with water.

- Let it rest within the refrigerator for round 2 hours without a doubt so the flavors and vitamins get infused.

Apple and Cucumber Fruit Infused Water

One important gain of apple and cucumber infused water is weight loss. Apples have numerous health advantages and beautify your popular health. Cucumbers have a large fiber content material material fabric which lets in in digestion. It can also help with precise stomach-related problems.

Ingredients

- three slices apple, halved

- 3 slices cucumber, halved

Instructions

- Mix the apple halves and cucumber halves in a box.

- Place them into an Acquablend basket making sure that they may be in identical quantities.

- Make nice which you do no longer fill extra than 2/three of the basket with fruit

- Now fill it up with water until the brim.

- Leave this mixture inside the refrigerator for at the least an hour or to permit for the approach of infusion to take place.

- You can choose out out to permit it stay within the fridge through the night time for added taste.

Blackberry Fruit Infused Water Recipes

Blackberry and pear fruit infused water

There are many berries and fruits which may be precise to the autumn season. You can revel in most of these stop end result with this drink. It especially includes blackberries and pears. Blackberries have low quantities of fats and calories. According to modern-day studies, additionally they help in improving cognitive abilities. Pears also have their non-public advantages. They useful aid in dealing with your weight.

Ingredients

- 4 Blackberries

- 2 pear slices, quartered

Instructions

- Take an Acquablend basket and location the berries and pear slices in it.

- Now fill it up with water.

- Let it relaxation inside the refrigerator for a few hours for infusion. Leave it within the fridge in a single day for more potent flavors.

Blueberry Infused Water Recipes

Blueberries and Orange Fruit water

This drink has a ton of health blessings. It is understood to reinforce someone's immune system. Blueberries are also believed to have sure recovery houses which might be very effective. This drink moreover improves skin circumstance and reminiscence strength. Oranges have a huge quantity of phytonutrients and weight loss plan C. They additionally consist of first rate portions of numerous distinct nutrients. They are rich in minerals along with copper and calcium.

Ingredients

- 5 blueberries

- 2 slices of orange, halved

Instructions

- Take a field and mix the blueberries and orange slices in it.

- Transfer this combination to an Acquablend bottle.

- Fill the Acquablend bottle with water.

- Let it rest within the fridge for some hours for infusion. Leave it in the fridge in a unmarried day for stronger flavors.

Creepy fruit infused water

This name might likely appear pretty absurd before the whole lot glance. It is a drink that is mainly made for Halloween. It is a amusing looking drink and is good for a Halloween birthday party. In addition to being a party drink, it tastes scrumptious and is distinctly nutritious and springs with some of fitness advantages. It is composed mainly of lychees and blueberries.

The 2 most critical components of lychees and blueberries are very wealthy in weight loss program C, which takes place to be a herbal antioxidant. They moreover consist of fiber and different vitamins that assist with digestion and moreover beautify metabolism of proteins, carbs and fats.

Ingredients

- 2-3 Lychee (peeled and pitted if smooth – or drained from tin)

- 2-3 large blueberries

Instructions

- Remove the seeds from the lychees. Now carefully insert the blueberries into those cavities on the manner to make something that looks as if "eyeballs".

- Put the ones "eyeballs" into an Acquablend bottle.

- Fill the bottle with water.

- Let it rest inside the fridge for a few hours for infusion. Leave it inside the refrigerator in a single day for more potent flavors.

Rhubarb Infused Water recipes

Cinnamon Rhubarb Explosion

Rhubarb is highly nutritious. It includes hundreds of vitamins, minerals, organic compounds and exceptional substances that help maintain our frame healthful. It moreover offers us with fiber. It aids us in weight loss and lets in prevent cardiovascular ailments. It will increase bone electricity and also improves the motion of blood. Cinnamon moreover allows by means of regulating the sugar ranges in blood.

Ingredients

- 1 stalk of rhubarb

- 1 small apple

- A stick of cinnamon

- Water

Instructions

- Cut the stalk of rhubarb into huge portions.

- Take the apple and wash it very well. Cut it into thin slices.

- Mix the ones substances in a subject after which switch them into an infuser bottle. Fill the bottle up with cold water.

- Now depart the aggregate inside the fridge for some hours and allow infusion take region. It is actually beneficial to head away it in a single day. Serve chilled.

Strawberry Infused Water Recipes

Strawberries & Mint

The strawberry within the water will artwork wonders because it has homes of being an antioxidant and an anti – inflammatory! It works toward preventing your pores and pores and pores and skin from sagging as properly!

Ingredients

- eight Strawberries (medium sized) sliced skinny

- four sprigs of mint

- ½ quart of water and ice

Instructions

Take an Acquablend bottle and place all of the materials interior. Add water to it. Let the aggregate stand for round an hour for infusion to take location successfully. Serve with ice.

Strawberry, Kiwi and Parsley Water

The elements of this drink are extraordinarily tasty. Most people love the flavor of kiwis and strawberries. This drink might be very fresh. Kiwis are very wealthy in nutrients C and E that assist in struggling with most cancers, developing antique and additionally enhance the immune device. They additionally include serotonin that has digestive and cardiovascular abilties. Serotonin moreover enables in regulating our sleep cycles. Kiwis also include a chemical known as lutein. This is a vitamins that combats eye defects which can be age related. Strawberries include anthocyanins that assist in reducing unwanted fat. They moreover sell bone energy and save you esophageal maximum cancers.

Ingredients

- 1 kiwi

- A cup of strawberries

- A few sprigs of parsley

- Half a lemon

- Water

Instructions

-Wash the kiwi and the lemon thoroughly. Cut them into very thin slices.

- Halve all of the strawberries. Place them in a subject on the facet of lemon and kiwi. Mix them properly.

- Transfer the contents into an infuser bottle. Add the sprigs of parsley. Fill the bottle up with cold water.

- You want not location this in the refrigerator for infusion, because it tastes specific no matter the truth that at normal temperature. However, it's miles better to serve the drink with ice.

Cucumber Infused Water Recipes

Cucumber & Lemon Medley

The cucumber on this water works as an anti – inflammatory and moreover permits in controlling the retention of water! Lemon facilitates in digestion and moreover continues you far from the not unusual cold!

Ingredients

- 3 cups chilled in spite of the reality that spring or mineral water

- 6 skinny slices of cucumber

- 2 skinny slices of lemon

Instructions

Take a container and blend the cucumber and lemon slices in it. Now add the water. Mix it well. Place in the fridge for as a minimum 2 hours for infusion to take vicinity. Leave in a single day for a richer flavor. Serve with ice cubes.

Citrus Cucumber Water

The cucumber on this water works as an anti –
inflammatory and additionally permits in
controlling the retention of water! Lemon
enables in digestion and moreover keeps you
far from the commonplace bloodless! The
oranges and the limes comprise Vitamin C that
lets in in cleaning your machine from the
pollution which could have accumulated.

Ingredients

- 2 massive lemons, sliced

- 2 massive limes, sliced

- 2 big oranges, sliced

- 2 large cucumbers, sliced

- 1 gallon of water

Instructions

Take an infuser bottle and upload the lemons,
limes, cucumbers and oranges. Fill it up with
water. Infuse in a unmarried day in the fridge.
Add the juice of 1 orange on the identical time
as serving for richer flavor.

Other Blends

Cherry Limeade

The cherries in the mixture and the lime have a
excessive quantity of Vitamin C that acts as a

first rate detoxification agent for the frame. You can be capable of clean your tool of any germs or antibodies.

Ingredients

- ½ Key lime, sliced thinly

- 3-pitted cherries lessen in half of

- ½ sprig of mint

Instructions

Take a area and mix the lime and cherries in it. Fill it up with water. Now add the mint. Place in the fridge over night time time for the flavors and vitamins to get infused. Serve chilled.

Pineapple & Mint Medley

Pineapple and mint are wonderful materials, which need to be consumed extra frequently for the purpose that you may be capable of clear your body of pollutants. You also can be able to raise your metabolism and your digestion.

Ingredients

- 2 pineapple slices

- 1 sprig of mint

- ½ quart of water and ice

Instructions

Mix the substances in an infusion bottle and fill with water. You need no longer vicinity this in the refrigerator for infusion, because it tastes accurate even if at ordinary temperature. Serve with ice.

Zesty Lime and Grapefruit Water

This recipe for infused water is especially glowing and is perfect for summers. The citrus stop result found in it's going to offer you with vitamins C and the drink itself will keep you hydrated. You can take a look at with masses of combos of the citrus end result and select them regular along with your possibilities.

Ingredients

- 2 limes

- 1 purple grapefruit

- 1 orange

- 1 lemon

- Water

Instructions

-Firstly, you'll want to halve the limes, lemon, orange and grapefruit. Now lessen the ones halves into thin slices.

- Now take an infuser bottle or beaker and location all the components in it. Fill it up with water till the brim.

- Now leave the mixture within the fridge and permit infusion take place. It is recommended to go away it in a unmarried day. Serve chilled.

Melon, Grape, and Honey Infusion

This is a few different drink that is quite clean and is proper for a hot day. The honeydew melons are candy and are wealthy in B complicated nutrients. Green grapes include massive quantities of nutrients and minerals and now have most cancers-fighting homes. The honey and mint are not only for which incorporates to the taste. They have anti-microbial and anti-fungal homes. In addition to those health benefits, the drink tastes without a doubt first-rate.

Ingredients

- 2 honeydew melon wedges

- 1 cup of inexperienced grapes

- Around 15 mint leaves

- Water

Instructions

- Take the honeydew melon wedges and do away with the center detail or center. Now lessen them up into small portions.

- Cut the green grapes in 1/2 of. Place them and the honeydew melon into an infuser bottle.

- Now upload the mint leaves as nicely. Add a small amount of honey for taste. Fill up with water.

- Let the mixture stand for round an hour or for infusion to take region efficiently. Serve with ice.

Tropical Coconut and Pineapple Water

Have you ever tasted a Pina Colada? This drink tastes approximately the identical so it's miles absolutely scrumptious. It furthermore has pretty some health benefits. Coconuts are appeared for their electrolyte content material and make this drink extremely smooth. The pineapple has massive quantities of magnesium and ascorbic acid. The drink continues you hydrated.

Ingredients

- 1 small pineapple

- 1 younger coconut

- Half a vanilla bean pod for flavor

- Water

Instructions

- Take the pineapple and reduce it down the middle. Remove the center. Now split the pineapple into bite-length quantities.

- Now take the coconut. Cut off the top component. Make a hole alongside the cut detail and pour out the coconut water into a tumbler (this may be used as a drink with the aid of the usage of itself). Remove the flesh of the coconut.

- Place all the substances in an infuser bottle and mix them a touch bit. Now fill it up with water.

- You want not vicinity this within the fridge for infusion, as it tastes accurate despite the fact that at ordinary temperature. However, it is better to serve the drink with ice.

Raspberry and Thyme Fusion

The additives of this drink are surprisingly rich in nutrients. Raspberries are specifically filled with masses of weight loss program B7, moreover known as biotin. Biotin has a number of beauty advantages. It prevents developing older, promotes smoother and softer pores and pores and skin, improves strength of hair and moreover enables in putting off scars of pimples or acne. The thyme offers a very characteristic taste to the drink and it also has excessive iron content material fabric.

Ingredients

- 2 cups of raspberries

- 1 cup of little one spinach

- 1 lime

- A few sprigs of thyme

- Water

Instructions

- Firstly, you will want to smooth the lime. Now reduce it up into skinny slices.

- Take an infuser bottle or basket relying on the quantity required (bottle for smaller portions and basket for big). Now upload the slices of lime, raspberries, cut spinach and thyme into the bottle. Fill the bottle up with bloodless water

- Place inside the refrigerator for as a minimum 2 hours for infusion to take vicinity. Leave in a single day for a richer taste. Serve with ice cubes.

Cranberry and Beet Water

The maximum crucial factor of this drink is the beetroot. It has a completely slight and exquisite flavor and is loaded with nutrients. It is specially rich in nutrients A (retinol), C (ascorbic acid) and D (calciferol). It furthermore has a large content material fabric of iron and calcium. The cranberries have a tart flavor and mix very well with the taste of the beets. This drink keeps you hydrated and is extremely smooth.

Ingredients

- 1 small beet

- A small quantity of beet vegetables (a handful will do)

- Half a cup of cranberries

- A teaspoon or of honey for flavor

- Water

Instructions

- Wash the beetroot. Now chop it up into skinny slices.

- Take an infuser bottle. Place all of the sliced beets, cranberries and beet greens in it. Fill it up with water. Add a small amount of honey. Do now not upload extra than 2 teaspoons or the flavor of the drink can be ruled via the honey.

- Leave this combination inside the fridge for as a minimum an hour or two to permit for the way of infusion to take area. You can pick out to permit it stay inside the fridge via the night time time for delivered taste.

Blueberry Chia Water

Chia seeds are stated if you need to absorb up to ten times their weight in water. They are rather wholesome as they are complete of nutrients. These vitamins may have important outcomes for your body and thoughts. The seeds have very low calorific content material material. The health blessings of blueberries have already been said before. This drink is incredibly clean and is ideal at some stage in summer time.

Ingredients

- Half a cup of blueberries

- Around a tablespoon of chia seeds

- One lemon

- A small quantity of honey for taste

- Water

Instructions

- First, take the lemon and wash it. Cut it up into skinny slices.

- Take a field and vicinity the blueberries, chia seeds and slices of lemon into it. Mix them nicely.

- Take an infuser bottle and add those elements on the facet of bloodless water. Add honey making sure that it does not exceed a teaspoon.

- Now go away the aggregate within the fridge for a few hours and let infusion take region. It is recommended to move away it overnight. Serve chilled.

Apricot and Purple Basil Water

The most crucial elements for this drink, as the call shows, are apricots and crimson basil. Apricots are loaded with antioxidants that help in stopping or stopping maximum cancers. Purple basil is thought to assist with the motion of blood. It can also combat insomnia.

Ingredients

- 2 massive apricots

- ½ a naval orange

- Around 10 or 15 purple basil leaves

- Water

Instructions

- Take the apricots. Wash them properly and reduce them in half of of. Remove the pits.

- Wash the oranges. Now lessen them up into skinny slices.

- Take a massive field and blend the apricots and oranges in it. Transfer the contents to an infuser bottle and fill it up with water.

- Let the aggregate stand for round an hour or for infusion to take region effectively. Serve with ice.

Black Forrest Cake Water

For this infused water drink, we use bitter cherries, coconuts and dates as the number one materials. It is stimulated by way of the classic Black Forrest cake. Coconuts are full of electrolytes and therefore this drink is highly easy. The sour cherries have a completely specific taste and moreover assist in enhancing pores and pores and skin fitness. The dates are sweet and function a flavor very similar to that of chocolate however they're wealthy in minerals collectively with potassium and magnesium.

Ingredients

- Half a cup of coconut flesh

- Three to four medium dates

- Around 10 bitter cherries

- A few drops of liquid stevia

- Water

Instructions

- Take the dates. Cut them in halve and pit them. Do the same with the berries as well.

- Take a box and blend the dates, coconut flesh and berries. Transfer the contents to an infuser bottle and fill it up with cold water.

- Add a few drops of liquid stevia. Place within the refrigerator for as a minimum 2 hours for infusion to take area. Leave in a single day for a richer flavor. Serve with ice cubes.

Plum and Persimmon Delight

Persimmons are quite nutritious surrender end result which can be wealthy in vitamins, minerals and vital anti-oxidants. Although the ones are pretty excessive in energy, they have got low fat content material cloth. They are high-quality property of fiber. Persimmons are especially wealthy in vitamins A and weight loss plan C. Purple plums are rich in various minerals collectively with magnesium, iron and potassium. Bay leaves (a similarly component) have a cooling impact at the stomach and moreover facilitate digestion.

Ingredients

- 2 small persimmons

- 2 pink plums

- A few sprigs of parsley

- 1 bay leaf

- Water

Instructions

- Take the persimmons. Wash and reduce them.

- Take the plums and wash them. Pit and halve them. Now take a container and add the ones to the box together with the persimmons. Mix the components.

- Transfer the contents to an infuser bottle and fill it up with water. Leave this combination in the fridge for at the least an hour or to permit for the manner of infusion to take area. You can select out to allow it live in the refrigerator thru the night for greater taste.

Passion Fruit Fresca

Passion fruit has a completely feature flavor that sticks out. It is every sweet and tart to flavor. It has some of health advantages. Some of those benefits encompass the prevention of cancerous increase, enhancement of immune function, development of eyesight, betterment of skin, law of blood pressure, enhancement of blood stream and advanced bone density. It additionally permits in stimulating digestion. The oranges and honey will upload flavor to the drink and moreover upload to the vitamins C content material fabric cloth. Parsley is used to feature freshness.

Ingredients

- 1 ardour fruit

- 1 naval orange

- A few sprigs of parsley

- Water

- A teaspoon of honey for flavor

Instructions

- Wash the oranges nicely. Cut them up into thin slices.

- Now, take the passion fruit and halve it. Remove the insides and add them to a box. To this area upload the orange slices as nicely and blend.

- Transfer the mixture to an infuser bottle and upload the honey and parsley. Fill the bottle up with cold water.

- Now leave the mixture inside the refrigerator for a few hours and allow infusion take region. It is actually beneficial to go away it in a single day. Serve chilled.

Bloody Mary Infusion

Bloody Mary is at the start a cocktail of vodka and tomato juice. This infused water drink is inspired via the cocktail. Needless to say, it has masses tons less strength than the real cocktail and does no longer include alcohol of any form. Tomatoes are a outstanding deliver of antioxidants and consequently assist combat maximum cancers. They have the capability to help alter blood pressure. Tomatoes moreover have excessive fiber content material fabric and might help prevent constipation. It tastes tremendous and is quite fresh.

Ingredients

- 1 tomato (cherry tomatoes will artwork as well)

- 1 stalk of celery

- A few drops of heat sauce

- A few sprigs of cilantro

- Water

Instructions

- Wash the tomatoes and celery stalk. Cut them up into sincerely thin slices.

- Place those into a box and mix them. Transfer the contents into an infuser bottle and upload the sprigs of cilantro. Add a few drops of heat sauce (relying on how quite spiced you want the drink to be).

- Add cold water to the aggregate.

- Let the aggregate stand for round an hour or for infusion to take location successfully. Serve with ice.

Blueberry, Cucumber, and Cilantro Water

Any berry infused water usually tastes wonderful and is tremendously easy. This drink can also permit you to shed kilos. The cucumber and cilantro assist in boosting metabolism. Blueberries are wealthy in vitamins and feature low strength. They have a totally excessive content material cloth of antioxidants. They moreover protect the ldl ldl cholesterol in the blood and DNA from getting damaged.

Ingredients

- 1 cup of blueberries

- 1 cucumber (preferably a smaller one)

- 1 lemon

- A few sprigs of cilantro

- Water

Instructions

- Wash the lemon and cucumber. Cut them into thin slices.

- Take a discipline and upload the lemon and cucumber slices to it. Transfer the ones contents into an infuser bottle. Fill it up with bloodless water and add the berries and cilantro sprigs as nicely.

- You need not area this in the fridge for infusion, as it tastes actual even if at ordinary temperature. However, it's far better to serve the drink with ice.

Berry and Sage Water

Berries are remarkable sources of antioxidants and as a end result assist in scuffling with most cancers. Also, they're enormously easy. Sage is an herb that has some of health advantages. It may be very effective in treating digestive troubles along side lack of urge for food, diarrhea and heartburn. Sage is likewise rather rich in copper, iron and weight loss program B1.

Ingredients

- 1 cup of blueberries

- 1 cup of raspberries

- 1 cup of blackberries

- Around 10 sage leaves

- Water

Instructions

- Wash all the berries very well. Place them in a subject.

- Now, add the sage into this area and slightly muddle it with the berries to intensify the flavor. Transfer this aggregate into an infuser bottle.

- Fill up the bottle with cold water. Place inside the fridge for as a minimum 2 hours for infusion to take place. Leave in a single day for a richer flavor. Serve with ice cubes.

Peach Cobbler Water

This drink is inspired via the traditional dessert of Peach Cobbler. It combines peaches and coconuts to offer a drink that tastes truely scrumptious. A peach is an incredible supply of weight-reduction plan C (an antioxidant) and might help fight most cancers. It moreover permits in improving preferred pores and skin fitness via way of making it smoother, eliminating wrinkles and scars of zits and acne. It additionally permits with enhancing the health of the coronary heart. Peaches are also rich in magnesium and potassium. As stated in advance, coconuts are storehouses of electrolytes and are very clean.

Ingredients

- 1 peach (ripe)

- 1 younger coconut

- A few drops of vanilla liquid stevia drops

- Water

Instructions

-Wash the peaches. Cut them up into very thin slices.

- Cut off the top of the coconut. Make a hollow in the lessen ground and pour out the water right right into a area and keep that in the fridge (this will be used as a sparkling drink through manner of itself).

- Remove the flesh from the indoors of the coconut. Put this flesh in an infuser bottle.

- Also upload the peach slices and a few drops of the vanilla stevia. Fill the bottle up with bloodless water.

- Leave this mixture in the fridge for at the least an hour or two to allow for the approach of infusion to take region. You can pick out to allow it live inside the fridge via the night time time time for extra taste.

Lemon Poppy Seed Infusion

When it includes the cooking enterprise, the combination of lemon and poppy seed may be very commonplace. Lemons have just a few electricity. They also are rich in pectin fiber, diet C, calcium and potassium. They additionally have antibacterial houses. Lemons are seemed to keep the pH degree of the blood and moreover help with digestion with the resource of promoting the producing of bile. Poppy seeds are exceptional assets of B complicated nutrients. Poppy seeds are rich in minerals like iron, copper, calcium, potassium, zinc and magnesium.

Ingredients

- 1 lemon

- A few poppy seeds (spherical 1 teaspoon)

- 1 or 2 teaspoons of honey

- four mint leaves

- Water

Instructions

- Wash the lemons well. Cut them up into very skinny slices.

- Take the slices in a subject and upload the mint leaves and poppy seeds. Mix them nicely. Transfer the contents of the field to an infuser bottle. Now add the honey and fill the bottle up with bloodless water.

- Let the mixture stand for around an hour or two for infusion to take vicinity efficaciously. Squeeze the juice of a lemon in even as serving to intensify the taste. Serve with ice.

Dragon Fruit and Grape Water

The dragon fruit is fantastically appealing to the eye due to its neon coloration. In addition to searching genuinely proper, the dragon fruit is particularly nutritious. For starters, it has low portions of ldl ldl cholesterol. It has terrific portions of nutritional fiber and antioxidants. It additionally permits in combating diabetes and developing old of the pores and pores and skin. The fruit furthermore suppresses arthritis. The crucial health advantage of crimson grapes is that they smooth up any brain unfavorable plaque. In addition to this, they guard the coronary heart and promote weight reduction.

Ingredients

- 1 purple dragon fruit

- A cup of crimson grapes

- 1 small cucumber

- Around 10 mint leaves

- Water

Instructions

- Wash the pink grapes very well. Halve them as speedy as they're dry.

- Peel the dragon fruit carefully. Cut the fruit into huge chunks.

- Wash the cucumbers as well. Cut them into thin slices. Transfer the slices right into a discipline and upload the dragon fruit and grapes. Mix them a piece and switch those contents into an infuser bottle and add water and mint leaves.

- Place within the fridge for at the least 2 hours for infusion to take area. Leave in a single day for a richer taste. Serve with ice cubes.

57

Chapter 5: Healthy Fruit Infused Water

Concoction

Citrus & Cucumber Water

Most people discover it hard to get via the summer season warmth with out indulging in fizzy beverages. The humidity need to get overwhelming especially in case you stay in a tropical america. Citrus end result like oranges and lemon contain a immoderate amount of nutrients C, that could detoxify the liver in addition to the digestive tract. The enzymes observed in citrus culmination moreover assist in growing your metabolism, for this reason breaking down the fat in your frame. Cucumber as an alternative acts as an anti inflammatory agent, thereby retaining your pores and pores and skin hydrated.

Ingredients

- 2 smooth oranges (sliced)

- Approximately 10 cups of everyday water

- 1 lemon

- 1 medium cucumber (sliced)

- four-5 mint leaves

Instructions

- Slice up the lemons

- Put the sliced lemons, oranges and cucumber in a huge pitcher at the facet of the mint leaves. Mix them nicely.

- Add 10 cups of water to the pitcher and blend nicely yet again using a large spoon.

- Place the pitcher within the fridge for at the least three hours for the infusion gadget to take vicinity. Leaving it within the refrigerator in a single day brings a rich flavor to it. Serve in big glasses with some ice cubes in it.

Watermelon and coconut cooler

Watermelon being in reality clean feels extraordinarily soothing amidst the scorching summer time warm temperature. High on anti oxidants, watermelon is known to be beneficial in fending off weight problems or coronary coronary heart diseases. Besides the health advantages, water melon moreover maintains your pores and skin hydrated for a long term and also allows in selling a healthy glow at the face. Also, coconut acts as a cooling agent while being immoderate on fiber and critical minerals. A perfect aggregate of candy and sparkling flavor, this purple cooler is tremendous to emerge as a staple in your home.

Ingredients

-4 cups of de-seeded and cubed watermelon

- four cups of coconut water

- 7-8 cups of ordinary water

- 1 sliced lemon

Instructions

- Place the cubed watermelon into an infuser.

-To it, add the coconut water, everyday water and blend nicely.

-Cut lemon slices and add them to the infuser. Stir properly for approximately a minutes.

- Let the mixture stand for no lots much less than hours for the infusion to take location. For higher results leave it in a single day in the refrigerator. Serve alongside facet ice cubes.

Peach Plum and Pear Infusion

As titillating because it sounds in your taste buds, this relishing drink is tremendous to maintain you glowing all day. Peaches are a wealthy supply of weight loss plan A, potassium and iron. On the other hand, plums consist of a immoderate quantity of fiber and sorbitol. The vitamins A observed in peaches and plums are quite beneficial for human eyesight. Pears are often recommended through dieticians for weight loss or for curing digestive troubles.

They moreover beneficial useful aid closer to danger of growing colon most cancers.

Ingredients

- 2 medium sized peaches

- 2 small plums

- 2 pears

-9-10 cups of water

- four leaves of mint

Instructions

- Wash and slice the peaches, plums, and pears and set them aside in a bowl.

-Transfer those slices to a big infuser collectively with the mint leaves. Mix them properly. Add three 10 cups of water to the infuser and stir nicely for about a minute.

-Let this mixture stand for approximately 2 hours in advance than serving. Alternatively, you may save it within the refrigerator for about 24 hours. Serve the drink with ice cubes.

Lemon Ginger detox water

The increasing rate of weight problems troubles nowadays motives humans to go overboard with weight loss diets. While maximum weight loss merchandise are being offered at outrageous costs within the market, a aggregate of lemon and ginger is specially effective similarly to mild for your pockets. Ginger, frequently used for weight reduction is also loaded with gingerols, a cleaning agent that consists of anti most cancers homes. The zesty lemon allows in flushing out pollutants from your body, at the same time as which incorporates a refreshingly tangy taste in your drink. This colorful drink is likewise a surefire manner to refresh your self fast with out which include some of energy in your food plan.

Ingredients

-7-eight cups of water

-1 medium sized ginger root (sliced or grated)

-1 lemon

-four mint leaves

-2 tablespoons of honey

Instructions

-Wash the lemon and reduce skinny slices

- Add the slices to an infuser collectively with sliced ginger root and mint leaves. Mix well.

-Add 7-8 cups of water to the infuser honey and stir well for a minute. Let the aggregate stand for 2-3 hours in advance than you serve, so it infuses properly. Storing this drink within the refrigerator for 24hours offers it a richer taste. Add ice cubes on the same time as serving.

Blackberry and Orange drink

These notable elements, blackberry and orange, make for a amazing concoction of flavors whilst being loaded with abundance of healing marketers. Packed with a excessive amount of nutrition C, they will be notably first-rate in flavor. Regular consumption of oranges and blackberries can keep your immune system bolstered and does wonders on your pores and pores and skin. Oranges are taken into consideration to be one of the healthiest stop result that would boost your energy degrees speedy. Colorful and rich in flavors, this concoction can also hold ulcers at bay.

Ingredients

-7-8 cups of regular water

-2 mandarin oranges

-1 cup blackberries

Instructions

-Wash the oranges properly and reduce them into thin slices.

-Add the ones slices to an infuser along side blackberries. Mix them nicely. Add some water to this combination and stir it nicely.

-When you allow this combination stand for two-three hours, it shall infuse properly.

-To extract richness of the culmination, keep it within the refrigerator in a single day. Serve the drink along aspect ice cubes. You also can enjoy at the fruit slices after you have have been given ate up the drink.

Blueberry and lavender drink

When it involves fruit infused detox water, we need to ensure to hold it thrilling. A daily dose of the identical detox drink can get silly and take the amusing out of the detox weight loss plan. Lavender petals can upload a excellent but diffused floral aroma to an in any other case boring detox drink. At the equal time, it's miles identified to have anti-inflammatory and antiseptic homes. Combine this with the pretty hydrating blueberries and you have an first rate concoction that makes your pores and skin radiant while flushing out all the bad pollutants from the body.

Ingredients

-1 cup glowing blueberries

-A handful of in shape for human intake lavender petals

-About 7-8 cups of water

Instructions

-Wash the blueberries nicely.

-Take a massive infuser and add the blueberries in addition to lavender petals to it. Ensure that the lavender petals are sparkling and properly wiped clean.

-Mix this drink nicely via using stirring it for about a minute.

-Leave this drink aside for an brilliant 3 hours for the infusion gadget to take region. A richer aroma may be obtained by using leaving this aggregate inside the refrigerator for an entire day. Always serve it with ice cubes.

Belly slimmer Strawberry and Basil drink

Curbing your urge for food can look like an uphill undertaking, particularly whilst you're on a weight reduction healthy eating plan. The commonplace starvation pangs can ship you right right into a frenzy, making it difficult to pay interest in your every day duties. Regular use of basil on your diet plan can depart you feeling fuller and energized at a few degree within the day. An dissatisfied tummy, not unusual hunger pangs, and fluid retention can all be taken care of by using using basil in your detox drink. Also, a handful of strawberries ought to upload a pleasant taste to the drink on the identical time as supplying a excessive amount of fiber vital for weight loss.

Ingredients

-4 basil leaves

-6-7 freshly picked strawberries (sliced)

- Half a cucumber (sliced)

- 10-12 cups of water

Instructions

-Wash the basil leaves and form of chop them.

- In an infuser, positioned the strawberry and cucumber slices on the side of the basil leaves and mix them nicely.

-Add some water to this combination and stir nicely the usage of a large spoon. It is vital to allow this aggregate stand for three hours for it to infuse nicely. Similarly, you could keep this mixture within the refrigerator and drink it at the least times a day.

-Serve this drink in a massive glass with some ice cubes.

Lemon and Berry detox water

Ideally, lemon want to be an important part of our each day meals. If your each day food plan does no longer consist of sufficient lemon, an appropriate manner is to use it inside the every day intake of fruit infused waters. The goodness of lemon inside the form of vitamins C performs a important characteristic in flushing out the pollutants out of your body. Packed with nourishing antioxidants, berries can extensively assist in accelerating your weight reduction regime. Drinking this thrilling concoction for about 12-15 days in a row on the side of a healthy healthy eating plan can come up with the an awful lot-preferred results on your weight reduction.

 Ingredients

-1 cup sparkling blueberries

-1 cup smooth raspberries

-1 sliced lemon

- 10-12 cups of water

Instructions

- Wash the berries. Ensure they're nicely wiped clean.

-Add the berries to an aqua combination basket on the facet of lemon slices. Give it a aggregate.

-Pour water into the basket and mix all the substances nicely with the aid of stirring it.

-Leave the aggregate in the basket for 3 hours earlier than you can serve. The longer you store this concoction you're certain to get a richer taste.

- Serve with ice cubes for that cooling effect.

Watermelon Rosemary Water

Avid dieters want to test extra with tropical stop end result like watermelon. More adventurous dieters ought to commonly need to feature a chunk of herbs in their detox waters. Rosemary can upload a candy odor on your drink, almost like a smooth cocktail. The combined flavor of rosemary with watermelon may want to make for a outstanding aggregate whilst retaining your body hydrated. This pleasant wonder can hold the boredom away close to your detox diet regime. Anyone who thinks alcoholic liquids are the most effective way to enjoy ought to offer this exceptional elixir a need to attempt.

Ingredients

- 2 cups of watermelon (cubed and deseeded)

-2 rosemary sprigs

-2 tablespoons rose water

- 7-eight cups of water

Instructions

-Gently rub the rosemary sprigs in among your palms so it releases the taste. Set aside in a bowl.

-Add cubed watermelon portions to the infuser. Pour water, rose water, and stir it using a timber spoon. Add the rosemary sprigs to it. Give it each distinctive stir

-Let the mixture stand for two hours after which serve. You can double up the amount of the additives and shop this drink the refrigerator for some other day.

-Ensure to serve at the element of ice cubes.

Strawberry, Apple and Cinnamon drink for adorable skin

One can in no manner undermine the significance of eating sufficient water to hold your pores and pores and skin clean and glowing. Dry pores and skin, pimples, acne and so on. May be decreased genuinely with the aid of ingesting as a minimum 7 – eight glasses of water every day. To this habitual, upload a bit of antioxidants and you'll have that more youthful glow to your face so you can leave you looking radiant. Strawberries and apples contain anti aging agent like biotin, which matches in competition to sagging skin. Cinnamon but, enables in enhancing blood circulate and maintains you sugar cravings at bay. It is also often applied in weight reduction diets. Adding a sprint of lemon zest to this drink ought to make it even greater fine.

Ingredients

-1 cup of glowing strawberries

-1 medium sized apple (thinly sliced)

-1 cinnamon stick

-Zest of one lemon

- 10-12 cups of water

Instructions

-Wash the strawberries nicely.

-Add them to a huge sized aqua basket. To this, add chopped apple slices, cinnamon and mix.

-Pour water, sprinkle a few lemon zest and gently deliver the aggregate a stir till it mixes properly.

-Now leave this aggregate in the fridge for some hours for the infusion to take location. You can save this mixture for some other day and consume as according to your liking. Serve it chilled.

Anxiety reliever Pineapple Strawberry drink

The idea of a strain relieving magic potion may additionally moreover furthermore appear like too suitable to be proper. However, this next fruit infused recipe is positive to go away you pleasantly amazed with its effects. Amidst the hectic schedule, place of job goers frequently prevent via the canteen to seize a cup of espresso. While coffee could surely look like a pressure reliever inside the 2d, more quantities of it can be harmful in your health. A fruit infused pressure-assuaging drink may be the proper answer you may be looking for. High in anti oxidants, pineapple, and strawberries may need to depart you feeling refreshed for the rest of the day. Slight little bit of apple cider vinegar may additionally help in weight reduction.

Ingredients

-Half cup peeled and cubed pineapple

-1 cup of strawberries

-2 tablespoons of apple cider vinegar

-7-eight cups of water

- 1 basil leaf

Instructions

-Wash the strawberries nicely

-Take a big pitcher and upload the washed strawberries to it. Now upload pineapple, basil leaf and mix nicely.

-Pour water into the aggregate. Add apple cider vinegar and deliver it a pleasant stir the use of a big spoon.

-Let it rest inside the refrigerator for a few hours so the aggregate receives infused nicely. Stronger flavors can be obtained if you depart it in a unmarried day. Serve chilled.

Blackberry and Sage water

The delectable aggregate of blackberries and sage may additionally need to make this drink one of the most not viable to withstand concoctions of all instances. The noticeably spiced sage can leave you with a experience of a complete tummy even as adding that an lousy lot desired area of know-how to this drink. This red coloured drink can effortlessly quench your thirst, at the same time as preserving you covered in opposition to acid imbalance, allergic reactions and reduces menopausal signs and symptoms. If you're feeling a piece extra adventurous, you can also attempt it with a sprint of mint or cilantro leaves.

Ingredients

-1 cup of glowing blackberries

- 4 sage leaves

- Few cilantro or mint leaves

-8-10 cups of ordinary water

Instructions

-Wash the berries.

-Rub the sage leaves the utilization of each hands and set them apart.

- In a huge vessel, add the berries, sage leaves, and cilantro and blend properly. Pour water and preserve stirring until it's blended properly.

-Transfer this mixture to an infuser bottle or a tumbler.

-Infusion system of this aggregate will take as a minimum more than one hours this drink may be stored for some unique day in the refrigerator.

-Ensure to serve alongside aspect a few ice cubes.

Kiwi lemonade

A delicious and juicy fruit like kiwi is one of the most perfect in phrases of making fruit infused waters. Having stated that, kiwi also can require a piece of greater soaking so it could release the most flavors. The splash of green color and the tangy taste can turn a smooth drink proper right into a more exceptional deal with. Since it's no longer bitter like citrus skins, you may moreover use the rind for brought taste to your drinks. The tangy flavor of kiwi and lemon may be balanced with a dash of honey and your drink is ready.

Ingredients

- 2 medium sized kiwis

- 1 sliced lemon

-2-3 tablespoons of honey

-7-eight cups of normal water

Instructions

-Wash the kiwis properly and cut them into thin slices.

-Take a big pitcher and upload the kiwi and lemon slices to it. Pour 8 cups of water, honey and stir properly.

-Like stated in advance, the kiwis may additionally moreover additionally take a piece longer to soak. Hence it's certainly beneficial to allow this mixture stand for 4 hours in advance than it's served.

-Ensure to feature generous quantities of ice cubes on the identical time as serving this drink.

Peach and Ginger infused cooler

I surprise if there may be something greater stunning than studying a e book on a lazy Sunday night time alongside a peach and mint cooler. This concoction can effects uplift your temper on the same time as supplying you with a cooling impact. The tasty peach is a superb snack for dropping those extra pounds. A unmarried peach consists of merely 50 strength without any fats. Plus, it allows in retaining your pores and skin healthful and hair loss at bay. A little little bit of mint in conjunction with some vanilla can beautify the taste of this drink with the aid of way of the use of some notches. If you don't find sparkling peaches, you can moreover use the frozen ones.

Ingredients

-5 medium sized peaches

- 6-7 mint leaves

- Half a pod of vanilla

-7-eight cups of water

Instructions

-Wash the peaches and slice them up the use of a pointy knife. Set apart.

-In a big infuser, add the peaches, mint leaves and mix.

-Pour water into the infuser and stir it. Add a piece of vanilla and offer it a stir once more.

- This concoction takes about 2 hours to get infused. Store it in the refrigerator for a few hours.

-Serve chilled.

Peach and Ginger Water

Take the warm temperature of the ginger and the splendor of the peaches, and you have an exciting drink that would quench your thirst without adding too many power. The numerous fitness benefits of every peach and ginger makes it for a high-quality health drink. It ought to comprise as little as 40 electricity constant with serving. You can add the peach and ginger skin to numerous deserts which incorporates cakes, panacotta or ice lotions for brought taste.

Ingredients

- 4 medium sized peaches

- 1 piece of ginger (2inch)

-4 sprigs cilantro

-7-eight cups of water

Instructions

-Wash the peaches and ginger nicely. Peel the ginger and reduce them into thin slices.

--Break the cilantro sprigs. Add them to a massive infuser. Now add the sliced peaches, ginger and mix.

-Pour water to this mixture and stir.

- Let it stand for 2 hours before you are organized to serve. You also can stress this combination earlier than serving. Alternatively after ingesting the drink you could additionally take pride in at the peach portions.

-Add ice cubes.

Cucumber and Lavender Water

This drink can assist in alleviating all varieties of indigestion issues, bloating, further to dehydration. Cucumber, diagnosed for its anti-inflammatory homes can provide a huge remedy for your tummy and help your body to rehydrate. The impact of lavender can useful useful resource in relieving tension or pressure issues, on the identical time as lending the drink a remarkable floral aroma. Adding mint to this drink can also ensure that you live smooth at a few level inside the day.

Ingredients

- 1 big cucumber

- 4-five lavender leaves (clean or packaged)

-5 mint leaves

-10-12 cups of water

Instructions

-Wash the cucumber and reduce it into thin slices the usage of a pointy knife.

- In a big field, add cucumber slices together with the lavender leaves. Gently rub the mint leaves the usage of every fingers and upload them to the combination.

- Pour water and stir the drink the usage of a huge spoon.

-Now switch this mixture to an infuser bottle and permit the infusion gadget take vicinity for about 2 hours. You can also refrigerate it in a unmarried day for higher results.

-Make sure to usually serve it chilled

Grapefruit, Mint & Ginger concoction

Grapefruits are considerably recognized to boom blood movement in the frame and works as an anti-growing older element. Regular use of grapefruits can not best sluggish down the growing old way but additionally treatments dry pores and skin troubles. Similarly, it's also mentioned to decorate the immune machine for that reason retaining you included in competition to illnesses. Most of our weekend hangouts go away us with a heavy hangover that takes a while to snap out of. This drink is exactly what you want to decrease the hangover in merely a couple of minutes of you eating the drink.

Ingredients

- 1 huge cup of smooth grapefruit

- Half a cucumber

-2 slices of ginger (2 inch)

- four mint leaves

-1 small orange (peeled)

- 10-12 cups of water

Instructions

- Wash and peel the ginger. Wash the grapefruit properly. Peel and slice the cucumber.

-Take a huge aqua mixture basket and upload the ginger slices, orange portions, mint and grapefruit to it. Pour a few water.

-Stir it properly the use of a wood spoon till it's mixed well. Leave this combination for three hours for it to launch most flavors. Store it inside the refrigerator if you would like.

-Serve with ice cubes.

Papaya and lime concoction

Papayas have located a place in a significant kind of cuisines all during the globe, especially Brazil and India. Papaya is packed with a excessive quantity of minerals, copper, and potassium which could lessen fatigue. Copper is idea to enhance the connective tissues in the frame and potassium can lessen the danger of coronary coronary coronary heart attacks. Papaya and lime collectively can assist in boosting your immune machine to a big quantity at the identical time as which includes scrumptious flavors to the drink.

Ingredients

-1 small sized papaya (ripened)

- 2 small sized limes

- Half teaspoon of vanilla extract

-7-8 cups water

Instructions

- Wash the papaya. Peel the pores and pores and skin off it and decrease it into small sized cubes. Cut skinny slices of lime the use of a sharp knife.

- Take a tumbler and add papaya and lime quantities to it. To this, upload the vanilla extract and pour water.

-Ensure to stir this combination properly so it blends properly. You can also use a few berries to provide it a tangy flavor.

- Let this concoction stand for 3 hours for it to get perfectly infused. You can continually store this drink inside the refrigerator for an afternoon. Be generous with the ice cubes while serving.

Mango and Mint cooler

Don't fear about no longer being able to discover a totally ripened mango. This drink can be produced from semi-ripened mangoes and however taste delicious. Mango isn't always most effective a scrumptious fruit but it's loaded with anti-oxidants. Also excessive in vitamins C, ordinary use of mango can play a important characteristic inside the production of collagen, that is beneficial in stopping the pores and skin from sagging. The special fitness blessings of mango embody cut price in ldl cholesterol issues, prevention in competition to most cancers and works in competition to night time blindness. Mango and mint makes for a soul soothing aggregate specifically while you feel worn-out.

Ingredients

- Medium sized mango

- 5 mint leaves

- 2 tablespoons of honey

-7-8 cups of everyday water

Instructions

- Wash, peel and reduce the mango into skinny slices.

- Take a large vessel and add the mango slices to it. To this, add mint leaves, honey and mix nicely.

- Pour water and provide it a stir. This particular drink can also need to be saved aside for 3 hours for the perfect infusion to take place.

- Serve chilled or use ice cubes.

Orange vanilla infused water

Orange blended with a dash of vanilla is a very healthy and a delectable concoction which also can be served in events. This drink may be a large hit amongst your own family and may be served along a few ice cream. Oranges are ideal for uplifting your mood without which include too many strength to your drink. Vanilla as a substitute, not best gives an oomph in your detox water, however additionally hydrates your pores and skin.

Ingredients

-1 massive sized orange

- 3/four teaspoon vanilla extract

-2 tablespoons honey

-7-eight cups regular water

Instructions

-Peel the orange and set apart in a bowl. To this, add honey and vanilla extract. Mix well.

-Take a big infuser and fill it with a few water. Add orange, honey and vanilla extract and supply it a stir.

- Allow this mixture to stand for an hour. You can also make this drink an afternoon beforehand of the birthday party and keep it organized for serving.

-Add ice cubes as consistent with your liking.

Cucumber and Jalapeno drink

If you have got been seeking out a kickass detoxifier, this drink is probably it. Slightly unusual mixture of the cooling cucumber with especially spiced jalapeno chilies is for the experimental dieters. Cucumber acts as a deterrent for kidney or liver issues, even as retaining the body far from ammonia. Jalapeno but can upload an on the spot oomph to maximum meals devices and is likewise recognised to reinforce up your frame's metabolism. The pretty spiced flavor of jalapeno chili may be adjusted in line with your taste. You also can spruce up the drink thru way of including a sprint of lemon to it.

Ingredients

-1 medium sized cucumber

-three small sized jalapeno peppers

-7-8cups of water

-Half a lemon

Instructions

-Wash the cucumber, jalapeno peppers, and lemon and decrease them into thin slices.

-Take a vessel and add the above additives to it and blend nicely.

-Pour water and supply it an incredible stir. Feel loose to modify the amount of jalapeno chilies used inside the recipe.

-Serve chilled or add some ice cubes to the drink.

Pineapple and Thyme water

Tired of the usage of the equal antique stop end result for making detox beverages? You should attempt at the side of a few herbs to make it thrilling. Herbs can turn a easy detox drink right into a flavorful and mouthwatering concoction you could't seem to get enough of. Pineapple consists of a blood-thinning agent referred to as the bromelain, thereby decreasing the risk of a coronary heart stroke. Whereas thyme can offer ample quantity of iron required in your frame to feature properly. It additionally alleviates infection and includes antibacterial homes. This sweet and herby drink is short to make and is amazing scrumptious.

Ingredients

-1 cup peeled cubed pineapple

-1 sprig of thyme

- 1tablespoon honey

-7-eight cups water

Instructions

-Rip the leaves of thyme and rub them slightly along side your hand for it to launch the maximum taste. Put it in a bowl and add pineapple quantities and honey to it. Mix all of the substances.

-Take a big infuser bottle and pour approximately 7-8 cups of water in it. Now add the mixture from the bowl, a spoonful of honey and stir for approximately some seconds.

-Set this mixture apart for 2 hours so it gets infused well. If you can't seem to finish off the entire drink, preserve it up inside the refrigerator for twenty-4 hours.

-Serve in appealing glasses.

Cranberry and Rosemary drink

We all are visible creatures when it comes to meals or liquids. The more appealing a drink seems. The greater we are interested in it. Some are so visible that they don't thoughts an attractive searching drink with a mediocre flavor. Here's a drink this is nearly picturesque in addition to tasty. Cranberries are an exceptional fruit to preserve your immune device healthy while offering you sufficient vitamins on the identical time. When you taste up the sweet and tangy taste of cranberries with a few fragrant rosemary, you get an amazing drink that could satiate your flavor buds.

Ingredients

-1 cup easy cranberries

-2 rosemary sprigs

-1 medium sized apple

-eight-10 cups of water

Instructions

-Wash the cranberries and apple. Slice up the apples the usage of a sharp knife.

-Rip the rosemary leaves for optimum taste. Add most of these substances collectively in a bowl and mix.

-Pour water in a large pitcher and upload all the materials within the bowl to it. Stir it nicely using a huge spoon.

-Infusion for this drink will take at least hours. Store it up in the refrigerator in a single day for a richer flavor.

-Serve chilled.

Cranberry, Orange & Bay leaf Cooler

If you're an avid fan of glowing tangy concoctions, this drink is for you. There are one in all a type techniques to convert apparently boring detox water into a flowery one. The combination of cranberry and orange plays out relatively in terms of flavors further to the colour. To upload an herby aroma, you could check with bay leaf to lend a unique taste to the drink. The phytonutrients found in cranberry guarantees that it's complete of antioxidants and acts as an anti-inflammatory agent.

 Ingredients

-1 cup of cranberries

-2 medium sized oranges (peeled)

-1 massive bay leaf

-7-8 cups of water

Instructions

-Wash the cranberries properly. You can cut up the cranberries to carry out greater flavors.

-Pour the water into a big discipline. To this, upload the cranberries, orange quantities, and bay leaf and stir nicely. Mix all the materials properly the usage of a massive spoon.

- Add a generous amount of ice cubes to this aggregate and leave it for infusion for 2 hours. Make this drink an afternoon earlier than the weekend so you can experience a comfortable middle of the night sipping on it. Store it in a unmarried day for twenty-4 hours.

-Go beneficiant with the amount of ice cubes at the equal time as serving this drink.

Apple and Ginger concoction

Apples have a much broader attraction in terms of its utilization in numerous precise substances. Besides its large utilization in desserts and juices due to the immoderate fiber content cloth cloth, it has numerous medicinal residences too. However, you have to be more cautious approximately choosing up the proper shape of apples from the marketplace. Always

89

test the apples for any wax coating they may be laden with, as they'll be sprayed with too many insecticides. Pick people who look genuinely red and function a non-clean cease. The super combination of apple and ginger may be a amazing treatment for cough too.

Ingredients

-2 medium sized apples

-2 ginger roots (2 inch)

-three tablespoons of honey

- 10-12 cups of water

Instructions

-Wash the apples properly. If you ended up searching for the wax-blanketed apples with the aid of way of mistakes, peel the pores and pores and skin off and reduce them into thin slices. Similarly, peel the skin off the ginger roots and slice them up.

- Take some water in an infuser. To this, upload the apple and ginger quantities. Mix them properly.

-Add a few honey to this drink and blend the factors well.

-Let it stand for 2 hours for the suitable infusion. Keep it inside the refrigerator for a few greater hours for a richer taste.

-Serve ice cubes with the drink.

Cherry and Mint infused Water

Going on a eating regimen can frequently leave humans with a sweet enamel yearning for sugar. While decreasing down subtle sugar out of your each day consumption is critical for weight loss, it can get difficult to control the craving. Cherries can upload that masses needed sweetness on your detox drink without which incorporates more power to it. Cherry and mint may want to make for a cute drink without added preservatives and chemical substances. The pepper minty taste of this drink can also even provide you with on the spot refreshment after an extended days artwork. Enjoy sipping it slowly with the aid of way of the use of the poolside on a lazy afternoon.

Ingredients

-1 cup of clean cherries

-five mint leaves

-Half cinnamon stick

-7-8 cups of water

Instructions

-Wash the cherries and reduce them into halves if you preference. Doing this can launch most taste and make your drink more relishing.

-Rip off the mint leaves and provide them a mild rub using your fingers.

-Take a large pitcher and add the cherries, mint and cinnamon stay with it. Pour water and preserve stirring it slowly until all of the additives get combined nicely.

-Leave it aside for two hours for the flavors to get infused. To get a richer flavor, preserve this drink in the fridge for about 24 hours.

-Add ice cubes whilst serving.

Mango & lemon grass infused Water

How about a lip smacking and thirst quenching cocktail minus the extra energy? It's a drink this is wealthy in flavors and at the identical time detoxifies your body. Using lemongrass for your detox waters can result in an X-element to an in any other case plain drink. Also, lemon grass can be grown for your personal nursery while not having a few detail else except a wealthy soil, strategically located pot in an effort to derive daylight hours and plenty of water. It facilitates in curtailing greater hunger; remedies water retention, and furthermore acts as an antioxidant that can prevent wrinkles from acting for your pores and skin.

Ingredients

-2 medium sized mangoes

-1 stalk of lemon grass (husk removed)

-5 strawberries

-10-12 cups of water

Instructions

-Wash, peel and slice the mangoes into small cubes. Similarly, wash the strawberries and decrease them into two halves. Set aside in a bowl. Bash the lemon grass barely so it releases a richer taste. Add it to the bowl and mix nicely.

-In a big aqua mixture basket, upload the components from the bowl collectively with a few water. Stir continuously for approximately a minute. Ensure all factors are combined well.

-Let this concoction stand for three hours in advance than it is able to be served. Doing this can allow the infuse way to take region. Refrigerate in a single day for higher flavor and taste.

-Add 3-four ice cubes in step with serving.

Blackberry and Lemon grass infused water

There's some thing nostalgic approximately sipping on a rustic drink from a groovy pitcher on a weekend campout, reminiscing all the great memories of your life. As enjoyable as it sounds, this drink can soothe your senses in mins and leave you feeling peaceful. This drink must your first-class savior on a blistery summer season morning. You can also integrate this drink with your each day cup of green iced tea. The aroma of lemon grass, tangy flavor of blackberry, cooling cucumber and revitalizing inexperienced tea can be truely what you need to kick start your day with a bang.

Ingredients

-1 cup of blackberries

-1 small sized cucumber

-1 stalk of lemon grass (de-husked)

-8-10 cups of water

Instructions

-Wash the blackberries and cucumber. Slice up the cucumber using a pointy knife.

- Bash the lemon grass stalk so it offers out a wealthy aroma.

-Fill some water in a vessel. To this, add the blackberries, cucumber, and bashed lemon grass and offer it a stir till all additives are mixed nicely.

-Transfer this combination to an infuser bottle and allow it stand for 2 hours. You can serve this drink together with some ice cubes after it has been infused properly. Alternatively you may keep it as much as 24 hours in the refrigerator.

Raspberry Peach and Kiwi water

Today an increasing number of humans are education themselves about the facet results of extra subtle sugar of their healthy eating plan. This reputation is supporting in ensuring that humans lessen down fizzy and sugary drinks from their weight loss plan. Fruit infused waters especially made using citrusy end result like raspberry and kiwi have become a huge hit amongst youngsters. Raspberry, kiwi and peach make for a glamorous looking drink that incorporates all of the trends of a fitness drink. This drink tastes slightly sweetish while no longer having to feature any sugar. Adding a piece of cinnamon to this drink moreover permits in accelerating weight loss.

Ingredients

-1 cup glowing or packaged raspberries

-2 small peaches

-2 medium sized kiwis

-Half a stick of cinnamon

-10-12 cups of water

Instructions

-Wash the raspberries, reduce them into halves if you preference. Wash the peaches, kiwis and decrease them up into slices.

-Take a big pitcher and fill it up with water. To this, add all of the end end result, cinnamon stick and stir till the components are combined properly.

-Let it stand for 3 hours. If you desire, you can refrigerate this drink for every other day. It will deliver out maximum flavors and make your drink even more thrilling.

-Serve this drink along with ice cubes on top.

Lime and Tarragon detox water

Not numerous people appear to increase a taste for Tarragon that without difficulty. However, if you use this herb reasonably and not permit it get overpowering, you are tremendous to get an thrilling aggregate of flavors. Tarragon is commonly used alongside citrusy end end result as it works nicely with them. Slightly anise like in flavor, tarragon is fine infused with lime. If you have never attempted tarragon in your detox water, it's approximately time you need to attempt it. This extremely fresh spa water may additionally even make sure that you stay a long way from fizzy drinks.

Ingredients

-2 medium sized limes

-half of cup easy tarragon leaves

-2 tablespoons honey

-7-eight cups of water

Instructions

-Wash and decrease the limes into skinny slices.

-Slightly bash the tarragon leaves for it to launch maximum taste.

-Fill up an infuser bottle with some water. Throw inside the tarragon leaves. Add lime slices to it alongside facet some honey and stir well for approximately a minute.

-Let this concoction stand for two to a few hours for the infusion to take location. Keep apart a few water inside the refrigerator so you can sip on it later.

-Serve along side a few ice cubes.

Banana Honey and Basil infused water

Bananas can also moreover look like an uncommon choice for making fruit infused waters for a few, however whilst you offer it a strive, you may want to use it frequently. A lot of humans assume eating bananas continuously outcomes in weight gain, but that's now not proper. When consumed cautiously, bananas can do wonders in your skin and fitness. They are immoderate in potassium and are widely identified to help proper digestion of food. Honey and banana can each hold your pores and skin hydrated for a long term. This sweetish drink with a slightly herby flavor of basil is sufficient to maintain your hungers pangs on top of things.

Ingredients

-1 big semi-ripened banana

-2 tablespoons honey

-2-three basil leaves

-7-8 cups of water

Instructions

-Peel the bananas and reduce them into slices. Set the slices apart in a bowl. To this, add a few honey. Gently bash the basil leaves and add them to the bowl. With the assist of a spoon, mix all of the components well.

-Fill up a pitcher with some water. Transfer all of the materials from the bowl to the pitcher and supply it a stir using a huge spoon.

- This mixture may additionally additionally take at the least hours to infuse. For better outcomes, store it up in fridge for twenty-four hours.

-Serve chilled.

Banana Pineapple and Mint infused water

If you in all likelihood did come to be liking the above-stated banana drink, you could love this one too. Here's a concoction that combines the hunger satiating homes of banana, the diet regime packed pineapple and the freshness of mint. As nutritious as this drink sounds, it's quite wealthy in taste too. Although you need to keep away from the use of greater ripened bananas as it could boom the sugar content material fabric of your drink. The cease result used to make this drink may also even supply an exquisite quantity of nutritional fiber for your body which essential for proper digestion.

Ingredients

-1 massive sized semi-ripened banana

-1 cup peeled and diced pineapple

-1 sprig of mint

- 12 cups of water

Instructions

-Peel the banana and cut it into thin slices using a sharp knife.

-In a separate bowl, add the sliced banana, pineapple and barely bashed mint leaves. Mix them together.

-Take approximately 12 cups of water in an aqua aggregate basket. To this, add all of the components from the bowl and preserve stirring until all substances are mixed properly.

-A minimum span of hours is needed for this drink to get infused well. For greater ideal flavor, attempt storing it up within the fridge in a unmarried day.

-Ensure to constantly serve this drink chilled.

Banana Strawberry & Cardamom infused water

Here's each other magical recipe which you choice you had tried your arms on earlier. Adding strawberry to your banana infused water makes this drink awesome tasty. Strawberries upload a stunning pinkish shade to the drink while giving it a slightly tangy flavor. Then we've have been given cinnamon that would make the drink effortlessly attraction on your senses and assist the detoxification machine too. Cardamoms are without problem available inside the marketplace and you may inventory them as a whole lot as 3 hundred and sixty five days in the refrigerator. Just make certain to keep them far from catching moisture.

Ingredients

-1 medium sized banana

-1 cup sparkling strawberries

-2 cardamom cloves

-10 cups of water

Instructions

-Peel the banana and chop it the usage of a pointy knife. Wash the strawberries thoroughly and slice them into halves. Add the ones additives to a bowl.

-Slightly pound the cardamoms for liberating its flavor. Now add it to the bowl and combined all the substances the use of a spoon.

-Take a massive pitcher and pour some water into it. Now switch the additives from the bowl into the pitcher and stir continuously for about one minute.

-Let this combination stand for at the least 3 hours for a richer flavor. You can choose to store this aggregate within the fridge for 12 hours for a splendidly infused drink.

-Don't forget about approximately to feature ice cubes on the equal time as serving.

Guava and Mango infused water

Guava is a few different fruit that most human beings don't don't forget including of their every day dose of detox water. The idea of the use of a fruit like guava may also moreover moreover seem barely stupid to you however whilst you combine it with citrusy cease result, it makes for a pleasing drink. Mango too works nicely with guava. Adding a spoonful of honey to this drink will best decorate the taste and supply it a pleasant aroma. You can as a substitute upload a clove of cardamom too if you would like. High in antioxidants and vitamins C, little do people recognize that guava protection dry pores and skin too.

Ingredients

-2 medium sized guavas

-1 semi-ripened small sized mango

-1 tablespoon honey

-7-8 cups of water

Instructions

-Wash the guavas and mango and chop them into small cubes. Put the ones portions in a bowl.

-Add some honey into the bowl and mix properly the usage of a spoon. Be positive to combination the combination nicely.

-Take a few water in a massive vessel. Transfer the substances from the bowl to the vessel and stir nicely. Pour this combination into an infuser bottle.

-To make this drink more flavorful, allow it stand for 3 hours or maintain it inside the refrigerator in a single day. Doing this could enhance the flavor of the drink.

-Add some ice cubes and serve this drink in attractive glasses.

Passion fruit Sage and honey infused water

Highly aromatic, best searching and citrusy, ardour fruit can turn out to be a proper away favored as regards to making your personal detox water. Most passion fruit fanatics can't appear to get enough in their everyday dose of passion fruit juice. Adding them on your detox water can provide you a big motivation to start taking area a wholesome eating regimen. For all oldsters which can be craving to give their diets a cheat day can without difficulty satisfy their candy tooth with the resource of manner of eating this detox water. The enormously spiced flavor of sage and the subtle aroma of honey can make you addicted to this drink

Ingredients

-2 medium sized passion fruit

-1 sprig of sage

-1 tablespoon honey

-7-eight cups water

Instructions

-Take the pores and pores and skin off of the ardour fruit and dice them up using a kitchen knife.

-Slightly bash the sage leaves for an stronger taste.

-In a huge infuser bottle, throw in the bashed sage leaves, cubed passion fruit, honey and blend the use of a large spoon. Pour a few water and offer this mixture a extraordinary stir.

-The infusion for this drink may additionally additionally soak up to a few hours. The greater time you save it within the fridge, the richer this drink shall flavor.

-Always serve with three-four ice cubes on top.

Passion fruit Rosemary and Chia Water

The citrusy passion fruit can taste even higher with a spoonful of chia seeds brought to it. Chia seeds can be taken into consideration to be one of the super elements which can immediately providing a cooling effect in your frame. Easily available in the stores and definitely cheaper, chia seeds as quickly as soaked can form a thin gelatin like layer round them just like tomato seeds. The sweetish fragrance of rosemary blends flawlessly well with the juicy ardour fruit, thereby growing a paranormal drink. Just make certain to keep away from over usage of chia seeds so it does no longer overpower the flavor of passion fruit.

Ingredients

-2 Medium sized passion fruit

-1 Tablespoon chia seeds

-1 Sprig of rosemary

-10 cups of regular water

Instructions

-Peel the pores and skin off the passion fruit and slice them up into small sized cubes the usage of a kitchen knife.

- You can each soak the chia seeds half of of an hour in advance for them to fluff up, or without delay throw in some at some point of the infusion approach. Rip the leaves of the rosemary sprig and gently rub it together collectively together with your hand to launch its aroma.

-Fill up an infuser bottle with a few water. To this, upload the ardour fruit slices, some chia seeds, rosemary leaves and hold stirring till it gets combined nicely.

-Letting this aggregate stand for as a minimum 3 hours will make certain proper infusion to take vicinity. Store it up if you would really like for every other 12 hours for a fantastic taste.

-Serve chilled.

Passion fruit and Kiwi infused water

A kickass combination of ardour fruit on the facet of some kiwi can be genuinely energizing. Not satisfactory does it make for a glamorous searching drink, however it also includes capable of get you comfortable in minutes after ingesting it. Both are highly juicy cease end result which could ensure a easy pores and pores and skin and higher blood drift. You can add any herb you would like to make this drink greater flavorful but the usage of a clove of cardamom seems like a extraordinary addition. If you pick a slightly sweetish flavor, you could additionally upload a spoonful of honey to this lovely concoction.

Ingredients

-2 small sized ardour fruit

-2 small sized kiwis

-2 small cardamom cloves

-7-eight cups of normal water

Instructions

-Take the pores and skin off the ardour fruit using a small knife or a peeler. Cut the ardour fruit and kiwis into skinny slices. Set them apart in a bowl.

-Slightly pound the cardamom cloves for releasing its aroma. Add them to the bowl. If you decide at the cardamom with out its pores and pores and pores and skin, you may use certainly the seeds.

-Fill up a massive glass pitcher with about 8 cups of water. Add the ingredients at the bowl to it and stir well the usage of a large spoon that may attain the stop of the bottom.

-Infusion method for this drink will take at least 3 hours. Give it some different 12 hours for an superior flavor and flavor.

-Use a beneficiant quantity of ice cubes at the identical time as serving.

Passion fruit, Tender Coconut and Vanilla water

Passion fruit and vanilla martini has been gaining hundreds of reputation these days. While an alcoholic drink can be sincerely thrilling at instances, sipping on some detox water using the equal combination tastes clearly as exceptional. This aggregate ought to make for a tremendous night drink, specially with the addition of gentle coconut quantities. While vanilla can upload a first-rate flavor to the drink, smooth coconut will offer you with that ice bloodless impact and leave you feeling with a entire tummy feeling. You also can gorge at the ardour fruit and gentle coconut slices after you've got fed on the drink.

Ingredients

-2 medium sized passion fruit

-1 cup clean coconut quantities

-1 teaspoon vanilla extract

-12 cups of water

Instructions

-Peel the pores and skin off the passion fruit the usage of a small knife. Cut it into small 1-inch cubes and set them aside in a bowl.

-Add the moderate coconut portions, some vanilla extract and blend well the use of a spoon.

-Take some water in a big vessel and fill it up with some water. Transfer the factors from the ball into the vessel and keep storing constantly for about a minute. Transfer this mixture into infuser bottles for storage.

-Let this concoction stand for three hours for the infusion approach to take place. Overnight storage of this drink inside the fridge is effective to make it more flavorful.

-Always serve bloodless or upload ice cubes on the equal time as serving.

Passion fruit, Papaya and Mint infused water

Passion fruit being barely tangy in taste, you may from time to time employer it up with a subtle flavored fruit like papaya. If you are a true ardour fruit lover, you can not want some different fruit to overpower its taste. This aggregate will stability each the flavors whilst you may satisfaction in on the fruit chunks after you finish off the drink. Mint is continuously a favorite amongst dieters nearly about their detox waters because it gives a sparkling taste to the drink while moreover assisting in smooth any digestion problems.

Ingredients

-2 medium sized ardour fruit

-1 small papaya

-2 sprigs of mint leaves

-10-12 cups of water

Instructions

- Take the pores and skin off the ardour fruit in addition to papaya the use of a kitchen knife. Cut them into small 1-inch cubes and set them aside.

- Slightly rub the mint leaves so as to get greater flavors off them.

-Take a few water in an infuser bottle. Add the papaya and ardour fruit cubes to it at the aspect of the mint leaves. Now cover the lid of the bottle and shake it for approximately a minute so all the materials get combined properly.

- Let this aggregate stand for two hours for the infusion machine to take location. Place it inside the fridge for a much flavorful drink.

-Serve in an appealing glass and upload some ice cubes.

Passion fruit Blueberry and cinnamon water

A lot of people with dry skin typically will be inclined to move berserk with splendor products to maintain their pores and pores and skin hydrated. While the usage of the proper moisturizer or each different beauty product can in fact do you some specific, it's moreover crucial to maintain the frame hydrated from inner. Adding citrusy end result on your daily weight loss plan guarantees a right blood float thereby maintaining your pores and pores and pores and skin hydrated. The greater hydrated your pores and skin stays, the better its possibilities of stopping it from getting dry.

Instead of spending a fortune on splendor products, you may use natural quit end result like passion fruit and blueberries to your weight-reduction plan.

Ingredients

-2 medium sized ardour fruit

- 1 cup of glowing blueberries

-1 cinnamon stick

-1 tablespoon honey

-12 cups of water

Instructions

-For starters, you need to take the pores and skin off the ardour fruit the use of a sharp knife. Cut them into small portions.

-Wash the blueberries. Add every the culmination in a bowl. To his, add honey and blend nicely.

-Fill up a few water in a large aqua aggregate casket. Transfer the additives shape the bowl to this casket and deliver it a stir. Add the cinnamon stick and stir all all over again.

-You also can switch this aggregate to an infuser bottle and permit it stand for 3 for it to get infused well. Alternatively, you may choose out to hold it in a single day in the refrigerator for a higher taste.

-Serve chilled.

Lychee and pineapple infused water

Who doesn't love lychees? This tropical fruit is effortlessly to be had inside the markets now. Fresh or packaged, it is able to add a top notch taste to a detox drink. Extremely rich in phytonutrients, antioxidants and vitamins B-complex, lychee also may be a lovable fruit to gorge on. This tiny searching fruit is likewise loaded with immoderate amount of nutrients that can be beneficial for your bodily abilties. The zesty pineapple brings a candy and tangy flavor to this drink and leaves you feeling satiated. A few leaves of thyme or sage may want to make this combination more exciting and keep the boredom out of the window as regards to detox drinks.

Ingredients

-12 medium sized lychees

-1 cup of cubed pineapple

-1 sprig of thyme leaves

-12 cups of water

Instructions

-Peel the pores and skin off the lychees using your hands. Remove the seed and reduce them into halves. Take a bowl and add the pineapple cubes and lychees to it.

-Rip the thyme leaves apart and gently rub them in between your fingers. Doing this can deliver out most flavor

-Fill up a massive pitcher with a few water. Transfer the components from the bowl to it. Throw within the thyme leaves and stir it for about a minute.

-Let the mixture stand for at the least 3 hours for a better flavor. For a richer flavor, shop this drink inside the refrigerator for another 12 hours and you are equipped to serve.

-Use loads of ice cubes on the same time as serving.

Lychee Orange and chia seeds water

Imagine sipping at the maximum rejuvenating drink in a spa on the identical time as playing the character. This particularly smooth drink is ideal for a hot sunny day. While it is blistering warm outside, you may experience comfortable and located your feet up at the same time as not having a factor to fear about. A wonderful mixture of lychee, chia seeds and orange can alleviate the extra heat in the frame. The punch of lychee whilst blended with the zesty orange can revitalize your senses without delay. The particular flavor of this fruit punch is advantageous to move away a cute aftertaste for your mouth the complete day.

Ingredients

-10 medium sized lychees

-1 medium sized orange

-1 tablespoon of chia seeds

-12 cups of water

Instructions

-You can without issue rip aside the lychee pores and skin the use of your naked hands. After peeling the pores and pores and pores and skin off, remove the seeds and reduce them into two halves. Set aside in a bowl. Peel the orange and add it to the bowl.

-In a large vessel, pour some water. To this, add the materials in the bowl. Throw in some chia seeds and hold stirring until it's mixed nicely.

-Allow this concoction to stand for three hours for a flavorful drink. Best results may be acquired by way of the usage of storing up this drink inside the fridge for twenty-4 hours.

-Serve chilled.

Lychee and ginger infused water

This combination may additionally seem unusual at the first pass, but we strongly endorse you to attempt it. The ginger root can convey a specifically spiced taste to the drink, which is precisely what you could want for the duration of a wintery middle of the night. When its winters, you don't need to gorge on too many cooling end end result as it can provide you with a cold. The cooling effect of lychee gets nicely balanced by way of which incorporates a few ginger to it. It might also additionally sound like an out of the sphere drink, however it could end up turning into your favored and moreover provide you with the medicinal residences of ginger specifically in winters. Ginger is also widely used for weight reduction beverages.

Ingredients

-12 large sized lychees

-2 ginger roots (1 inch every)

-1 tablespoon honey

-12 cups of everyday water

Instructions

-Wash the lychees and rip its pores and pores and skin aside. Cut them into halves the use of a kitchen knife.

-Wash the ginger roots nicely. Ensure it's no longer muddled with soil. Peel its pores and skin off the usage of a peeler. Cut into thin slices.

-To a big pitcher, upload some water together with the above materials and mix nicely. Add a spoonful of honey and deliver it a tremendous stir.

-Allow this combination to get infused for approximately three hours. You can also switch this liquid in an infuser bottle and preserve it inside the ridge in a unmarried day.

-Serve together with a few ice cubes on top.

Dragon Fruit coconut water and basil concoction

While all people agree that taste topics the maximum in preference to how the food or the drink appears, permit's admit it, I ought to choose an splendid searching drink. Dragon fruit makes the drink visually lovely at the identical time as including its sparkling and unique flavor to it. This pinkish magenta colored drink is a few difficulty all and sundry wants to gorge on at house events. Since kids are extra seen, they may experience this drink the maximum. Basil is applied in severa from of cuisines to beautify the flavor the meals. Using Basil detox water enables in cleaning your digestive tract and could boom blood circulate.

Ingredients

-2 medium sized dragon fruits

-2 huge cups of coconut water

-6 basil leaves

-12 cups of water

Instructions

-Using a small knife, make an prolonged slit at the skin of the ardour fruit. Now rip off the pores and skin the use of your palms and take away the fruit. Cut it into small cubes and set it apart.

- Take an infuser bottle and fill it up with some water. To this, add a few coconut water, basil leaves, ardour fruit cubes and close to the lid of the bottle. Now provide it a pleasing shake so all of the materials within the bottle mix nicely.

-Allow this aggregate to get infused within the bottle for more than one hours. Store this bottle within the refrigerator if you need a richer flavor.

-Don't forget about to add a generous quantity of ice cubes at the same time as serving this drink.

Dragon fruit lemonade

Are you making plans on selecting up lemonade bottles from Wal-Mart for that football wholesome you're making plans to ask your buddies for? Soda based totally drinks really double up your leisure, however one doesn't apprehend how badly it affects your health. Instead permit's attempt a detox drink that might be genuinely as smooth, healthy and certainly delicious too. Lemonade can provide that immediately splash of strength you want at the equal time as proving to be extremely healthful on your body. You can add a bit of pomegranate and upload a more sweetish flavor to the drink. Dragon fruit lemonade isn't a few component that has been experimented sufficient regardless of its palette soothing taste.

Ingredients

-2 medium sized dragon fruit

-2 medium sized lemons

-1 small cup of pomegranate (peeled)

-12 cups of water

Instructions

-Rip the pores and skin off the dragon fruit thru developing a slit on it using a knife. It's smooth to drag aside the pores and skin the usage of your arms. Now reduce the ardour fruit into small cubes.

-Wash the lemons and decrease them into thin slices

-Add water to a big pitcher. Throw within the dragon fruit quantities on the facet of the lemons. Add pomegranate seeds and use a massive spoon to stir this aggregate. Ensure to stir it for some time so all factors get blended properly.

-Serve chilled.

Dragon Rosemary and Watermelon drink

The very attractive looking dragon fruit isn't handiest a visible address however additionally consists of severa health blessings. The cactus like pores and skin of the dragon fruit resembles almost like a legendary dragon, as a result the decision "dragon fruit". This tropical fruit can be placed in abundance specially in Asian nations as well as South America. Regular use of dragon fruit in your food regimen lets in in preserving your cardiovascular fitness affords you sufficient quantity of fiber fights blood sugar issues and lowers the signs and symptoms and signs and symptoms of growing vintage. Watermelon and dragon are both excessive of their antioxidant houses and make for a delectable drink.

Ingredients

-2 medium sized dragon fruit

-1 large cup of watermelon (pores and pores and skin eliminated and cubes)

-1 sprig of rosemary

- 12 cups of water

Instructions

-Take the pores and pores and pores and skin off the dragon fruit. Due to its thin pores and pores and skin, you can without problems peel it through creating a slit. Now cut the fruit into small 1-inch cubes.

- To a bowl, upload the watermelon and dragon fruit quantities and set apart. Slightly rub the rosemary leaves to release its flavor and add it to the bowl. Mix properly the use of a spoon.

-Add some water to a large pitcher. Add the combination from the bowl and the usage of a big spoon preserve stirring it until combined well.

-Let this concoction stand for about 3 hours for the infusion to take location. If you want to keep this drink maintain it within the refrigerator in a unmarried day. This may moreover beautify its flavor.

-Serve chilled.

Pomegranate and Cucumber drink

Staying hydrated does not need to be dull or which you need to drink gallons of normal water. Ideally, your water intake desires to be as a minimum 6-8 glasses in your body to feature well. But why make this a monotonous habitual on the same time as you can use interesting mixture of pomegranate and cucumber on your detox drink. Pomegranate is notion to have one of the most quantities of antioxidants content cloth amongst stop end result. These purple pearls are highly useful in doing away with any tummy problems or bloating. By combining the candy juice taste of pomegranate and the cooling cucumber, you get a superb summer time drink.

Ingredients

- 2 cups of pomegranate (pores and skin eliminated)

-1 medium sized cucumber

- Zest of one massive lemon

-10-12 cups of water

Instructions

-Wash the cucumber and decrease it into skinny slices.

-In a bowl, add the pomegranate, cucumber slices, lemon zest and mix the use of a spoon.

-Pour a few water in a large infuser bottle. To this, add the elements from the bowl. Close the lid of the bottle and shake it for some seconds so the concoction gets mixed well.

-Serve chilled

Pomegranate Ginger and Limewater

Planning an all female's night time day trip on a wintery middle of the night? Ditch that cola for this top notch tasty detox drink with out which includes extra energy. This ideal thirst quencher is a incredible preference on a chilly night time surrounded with the aid of the use of friends. The candy taste of pomegranate on the facet of a few juicy lime and highly spiced ginger will make you need to sip on it the complete day.

Ingredients

-2 cups of pomegranate (peeled)

-1 -inch ginger root

-1 medium sized lime

-12 cups of water

Instructions

-Wash the ginger root and lime properly and reduce them into skinny slices. Set them aside in a bowl.

-Add pomegranate to the bowl and mix the usage of a spoon.

-Fill up a pitcher with regular water. Now transfer the components from the bowl and provide it a wonderful stir using a wood spoon.

-Now that your mixture is ready, you want to allow it to stand for 3 hours. For a higher taste, go away it in a single day inside the fridge.

-Serve on the aspect of ice cubes.

Chapter 6: My Fruit Infused Water Recipes -

Just Add Water!

The water recipes in this book are all beneficial on your not unusual health and well-being. There are over 50 of them and they may be in no particular order of significance. I virtually have honestly put together as a set of my favored liquids that I want to make.

I honestly have included some useful records approximately the vitamins and minerals which is probably present in the end end result and herbs used inside the individual recipes in addition to statistics about what each drink is right for health sensible. This is for your records handiest and isn't supposed to be regarded as professional medical advice. Feel unfastened to research in addition the particular health benefits of man or woman end cease result, herbs and spices to appearance how they'll gain you within the long time.

With that stated, proper right right here are my preferred recipes.

1. Blueberry Orange Cooler

2. Cucumber Detox Water

three. Pomegranate & Blueberry Combo

four. Orange, Lemon & Lime Tonic Water

five. Pineapple, Orange & Ginger Breeze

6. Peach & Peppermint Healing Water

7. Lemony Lavender Life Saver

8. Strawberry Pineapple & Cinnamon Booster

9. Watermelon & Rosemary Water

10. Kiwi & Coconut Infused Water

11. Cherry Mint Health Booster

12. Green Lemonade Tonic Water

thirteen. Deep Berry Infused Water

14. Cucumber & 3 Citrus Water

15. Pineapple & Mint Refresher

16. Raspberry & Lemon Infused Water

17. Watermelon Cooler

18. Mango & Mint Infused Water

19. Melon & Strawberry Infused Water

20. Orange & Grapefruit Infused Water

21. Lemon Strawberry & Basil Blast

22. Apple & Cinnamon Infused Water

23. Grape & Melon Infused Water

24. Raspberry, Peach & Kiwi Water

25. Blackberry & Sage Infusion

26. Apple, Strawberry & Lemon Mint Water

27. Mango & Strawberry Cooler

28. Orange & Mint Infused Water

29. Apple, Pineapple & Cucumber Infused Water

30. Strawberry & Lemon Water

31. Raspberry & Lime Water

32. Iced Ginger Water

33. Fennel & Lemon Water

34. Green Tea, Lime & Mint

35. Watermelon & Basil Infusion

36. Orange, Lime, Strawberry & Lemon Infusion

37. Strawberry & Mint Booster

38. Lime & Cherry Infused Water

39. Kiwi Spa Tonic

forty. Watermelon Hydrating Water

forty one. Orange & Rosemary Infusion

forty . Coconut & Lime Infused Water

forty three. Raw Cucumber Infusion

40 four. Lemon, Blueberry & Mint

45. Simple Strawberry Infused Water

forty six. Blackberry & Mint Infused Water

47. Cranberry & Apple Classic

forty eight. Skinny Lemon Infusion

forty nine. Orange & Ginger Infusion

50. Triple Berry Infused Water

51. Aloe Vera Water of Life

fifty . Strawberry, Vanilla & Basil Infusion

fifty 3. Lime & Ginger Infusion

Pick a few difficulty that sounds right to you and let's get started out!

Basic Set up & Equipment Needed For Making Fruit Infused Water

The fantastic component about making fruit infused water is which you honestly most effective need simple device to get started. You will probably have most of this already. You will want:

•   Glass pitcher (or you may use mason jars) or any bottle with a substantial top

•   Strainer (for straining juice to take away bits/pulp)

•   Sharp knife (for slicing fruit)

•   Water bottles (for decanting water)

As well because the system listed above, you excellent need to have some clean or frozen give up stop end result of your desire, some herbs and a few spices.

That's it absolutely. There's now not whatever fancy approximately it. No excuses, you just need to get commenced. Find a recipe you need and offer it a strive. You will discover it impossible to face up to and your body will thank you for it too.

Some Major Health Benefits - Why Water Is So
Important

There are such numerous number one health
benefits related to consuming easy water on its
personal but; you could add herbal sparkling
fruit and herbs to water to advantage even
more fitness benefits. This now not only
improves the taste of the water, it additionally
guarantees essential nutrients are being located
into your gadget.

Drinking more water may be very vital for the
proper protection and care of our our bodies.
Water lets in with:

- Aiding your digestive tool

- Helping to suppress your urge for food

- Helping to govern and stabilize your weight

- Flushing out pollutants out of your frame

- Hydrating your body

- Enhancing your hair and pores and pores
and skin

To call but the numerous blessings. My belief is which you could as properly make your own fruit infused water at domestic so that you can control what you're doing. The hold supplied waters aren't only highly-priced, maximum of them additionally include delivered preservatives, nasty sugars as well as synthetic sweetener and shades. Next time you choose out a bottle of flavored water up, take a look at the listing of factors on the label. You might be taken aback.

Besides understanding exactly what you're setting into your body (even as you make your non-public) fruit infused water is likewise a awesome possibility to coffee and one among a type caffeine laced beverages that you may be tempted to have for the duration of the day.

If you have youngsters like me this is another real reason to begin introducing fruit infused water into your healthy dietweight-reduction plan. Your children will advantage from it the maximum and it is a splendid way of making sure they may be consuming sufficient water subsequently in their day. My kids love fruit infused water and each (I honestly have three) has their non-public desired. They even make it themselves.

Why You Need More Water Inside You - 10 Reasons To Consider

The simple truth is that consuming water is right for you. I may additionally want to forestall right proper here and depart the rest of this bankruptcy easy due to the truth that sentence summarizes the whole thing that you want to recognize. Although there is a lot of mixed advice around exactly how a whole lot water to drink on a daily basis, it is recommended that 6-eight glasses is prepared right.

Plain and easy, water is like gasoline for your body. If we liken our bodies to vehicles in the identical way that oil is vital for the inexperienced on foot of a car, the better oil you use on your car, the higher the engine will perform and your car will remaining longer too. Try to run your automobile without collectively with any oil and you may see the damage this will reason. It's the equal with the frame. You need to gasoline it with the proper fluid so as for it to carry out at its maximum effective degree.

TEN GOOD REASONS WHY YOU NEED MORE WATER INSIDE YOU:

1. Drink water or die. Drastic I recognize but it simply is the reality. Do that we can't continue to exist very extended with out water and can in truth stay to tell the tale an entire lot longer without food? If this is the case, why do most people devour plenty meals then and drink such little water? It is the sign of the times I guess. Fact is the greater water you drink the healthier you becomes.

2. Helps maintain frame moisture. Without water your frame is suffering. Water is needed for the important and effective functioning of your eyes, nose, mouth, mind, blood, bones and joints.

3. We are product of 60-70% water. It makes best experience then that with the intention to hold appropriate health, we want to pinnacle up our herbal water financial institution on a every day basis.

4. Drinking water aids digestion, waft and the renovation of your body temperature. Essential to life, improved consumption can cause higher physical, mental and emotional health.

5. Drinking water promotes weight loss - We all eat an excessive amount of sometimes however while you start to drink extra water, you will enjoy entire for longer and consequently reduce your calorie intake on a every day foundation. The vicinity of eating water continuously additionally permits to inform your mind which you have determined on a more fit way of life. Eventually you can start to crave water (in choice to the sweet and really risky soda beverages, coffee and alcohol).

6. Gets rid of pollution - The nasty increase of pollution can be unstable to your frame. Water helps to flush them out of your device. You launch greater pollutants thru your sweat glands and because of the fact you may be going to the relaxation room greater, you may launch greater pollution the greater water you drink.

7. Nature's final anti-age remedy - Water genuinely does assist prevent aging. Drinking more could wipe years off how you appearance. A herbal moisturizer, water lets in to maintain

pores and pores and skin looking greater younger, softer and wrinkle loose for longer.

8. Controls your mood - Yes it's far real. It is stated that thru consuming greater water and in the end improving hydration, you can decorate your feeling of fitness and your mood. You will experience much much less traumatic and careworn and further capable of deal with the traumatic conditions you face each day.

9. Combat Fatigue - Tiredness and dehydration drift hand in hand. When your body is dehydrated, you could revel in complications and expanded tiredness. This way that your cells aren't getting the nutrients it desires to hold you feeling your fantastic. The increase of water for your food plan

10. Calorie Free - Water consists of no strength so there can be no fear that you may advantage weight.

Plain Water Is Boring! Why You Need To Drink These Fruit Infusions Instead & FAQ's

Some humans like smooth antique silly water however I am no longer one in every of them! I surely did not drink enough water in advance than I started out out to introduce fruit infused water into my food plan and neither did my husband or kids. Since then we do not conflict to hold up with our water intake. It has grow to be a pride.

There are actually masses of various fruit and herb infused water combos to strive. After checking out some of the recipes in this e-book, you may absolute confidence provide you with masses of latest recipes of your very very own as nicely. That is the beauty of introducing this new manner of eating water into your life. It makes you come to be extra creative within the kitchen.

What Type Of Water Do I Use?

I use herbal spring or mineral water but you may use any kind that you like. You also can even use undeniable faucet water (boil it and allow it to take a seat back first) in case you do not need to go to the value of buying water.

The intention right right here is not to get right proper right into a debate about what sort of water is the exquisite. Just be confident that they'll be all pretty masses OK and will benefit you in some manner. If you are very particular in phrases of eating water, you could comprehend what type is excellent to suit your goals for every recipe.

Most of the recipes in this ebook point out herbal spring or mineral water so truely update this with the water of your preference.

Do I Adapt These Recipes At All?

Yes, I adapt the recipes in this e-book if I do no longer need to make up a ordinary sized pitcher of infused water. If I need to make the ones recipes in mason jars then I certainly lessen the amount of fruit and herbs therefore and check with the quantities until I get a taste that I love. You can do the same.

I am moreover constantly trying considered one among a kind fruit/herb combos to look how they flavor and what effect they've got on me and my frame. All the stop result which are listed in this e-book are conveniently to be had in maximum places but in case you can not find a specific fruit, then you can sincerely alternative it with a fruit of your desire.

Don't allow the simplicity of those fruit infused water recipes fool you. What is each accurate and critical approximately those recipes isn't always most effective the simplicity in putting them together however furthermore the mixture of the stop result and herbs and the impact that they've on fitness and healing while used collectively.

These fruit infused waters have helped me to kick my caffeine addiction and candy cravings which added about over 20lbs in weight reduction over a six week length. I now have fewer aches and pains, I without a doubt have got rid of my irritable bowel troubles, I sense top notch and I usually have a more amazing outlook on existence.

Do I Always Use Fresh Fruit?

No, I frequently use frozen culmination. Frozen give up result are not as lousy as humans on occasion make out. Much of the frozen fruit that we can buy has been frozen inside hours of it being picked therefore retaining most of the important vitamins in the fruit. For this cause, I do now not have a problem using it. If the recipe on this e-book calls for clean stop cease result, you can replace people with frozen if you have them.

How Long Does Fruit Infused Water Last?

I actually have found that I can keep my water within the fridge for up to two days (topping it up with smooth water at the same time because the pitcher is walking low). After this time, maximum of the juices will were infused into the water and it does no longer taste as extreme because it did as quickly as I first made it. The water also can become cloudy in appearance due to all of the sediment from the fruit that has constructed up inside the pitcher.

These fruit infused waters are so clean to make that it takes approximately 5 minutes to make up a sparkling batch so that you in no manner need skip without. As prolonged as you have some sparkling or frozen culmination and herbs then you will be able to make it as and at the same time as you please.

What Else Do I Do With The Fruit?

As well as making fruit infused water, I frequently make up a batch of ice cubes with a bit of fruit and sprig of herb in every one. These fancy ice cubes supplement your liquids highly and additionally appearance quite in particular if you have visitors over that you want to have an effect on. Try some of the ones, they're extraordinary and you are quality limited with the aid of your very own imagination in terms of the extremely good fruit cube combos which you provide you with.

So now that you have the vital rundown on a number of bits and bobs of my fruit infused water endeavors, skip over to the recipes and try some of them. Stick to the world of consuming awesome waters on a regular foundation (it is endorsed that we consume about 6-eight glasses an afternoon) and you too will word which you start to take manipulate over any urges you have got had been given for those sweet soda liquids which may be so especially lousy for you. Your caffeine addiction (if you have one) can have with a bit of luck subsided too.

Blueberry Orange Cooler

Active Minerals: Potassium, Calcium, Iron, Zinc

Active Vitamins: A, B complex, C, E, K

Other Facts: Low in electricity, natural anti-oxidant

Good For: Helps restriction loose radicals within the body, complex nutrients help the frame metabolize carbs, protein and fat.

Ingredients

• 6 cups water

• 2 mandarin oranges (reduce them into quarters)

• Handful of blueberries

• Handful of Ice

Directions

1. Place the mandarins and blueberries in a tumbler

2. Mash the fruit barely to release the flavor and infuse the water

three. Add water and ice

four. Let it sit within the refrigerator for two-four hours earlier than serving

5. Enjoy your delicious healthy drink

Cucumber Detox Water

Active Minerals: Potassium, Calcium, Magnesium

Active Vitamins: A, B1, B2, B6, C, E, K

Other Facts: Cucumber includes Silica which promotes bone health. Citrus fruit full of important vitamins and minerals

Good For: Re-hydration and detox, particular pores and pores and skin and hair, weight loss & digestion. Also stated to reduce horrible breath.

Ingredients

- 6-8 cups natural spring water
- 2 large lemons (lessen into slices)
- 1 huge orange (reduce into slices)
- 1/2 of cucumber (reduce into slices)
- A few sparkling mint leaves
- Handful of Ice

Directions

1. Place the lemons, orange and cucumber in a pitcher
2. Mash barely to launch the flavor
3. Pour the water over it
4. Let it take a seat within the fridge for two-four hours in advance than serving
5. Serve in tall glass with ice
6. Enjoy your scrumptious healthy drink

Pomegranate & Blueberry Combo

Active Minerals: Potassium, Magnesium, Phosphorus, Calcium

Active Vitamins: B1 B2 B6 C E K

Other Facts: Pomegranate is one of the oldest seemed give up quit result

Good For: A compound this is decided best in pomegranates referred to as Punicalagin is shown to advantage the coronary coronary heart and blood vessels. Blueberries assist remove free radicals from the body

Ingredients

- 6 cups water
- Handful of blueberries
- 2 cups pomegranate seeds
- Handful of Ice

Directions

1. Place the blueberries and pomegranate seeds in a tumbler

2. Cover and allow it sit down for no a whole lot less than 2 hours (four-6 hours works terrific)

three. Add water and ice

four. Enjoy your scrumptious wholesome drink

Orange Lemon & Lime Tonic Water

Active Minerals: Potassium, Phosphorus, Calcium, Magnesium

Active Vitamins: A, B1 B2 B6 C E

Other Facts: Rich in nutritional fiber and entire of vital vitamins and minerals

Best use: Good anti-oxidant drink

Ingredients

- 6-8 cups herbal spring water
- 1 massive orange (sliced)
- 1 big lemon (lessen into quarters)
- 1 massive lime (reduce into quarters
- Small handful of cilantro

Directions

1. Place the orange, lemon, lime and cilantro in a pitcher

2. Slightly mash the fruit to release the taste and infuse the water

3. Add water and ice

4. Let it sit down within the refrigerator for two-4 hours earlier than serving

5. Serve in tall glasses with ice

Pineapple, Orange & Ginger Breeze

Active Minerals: Potassium, Magnesium, Phosphorus, Calcium

Active Vitamins: B1 B2 B6 C E K

Other Facts: Excellent anti-oxidant

Good For: Digestion and improved motion. The ginger is also diagnosed to be nicely for morning sickness.

Ingredients

- 6-eight cups natural spring or mineral water
- 1 small clean pineapple (crushed)
- 1 medium duration orange (sliced)
- 2 tablespoons freshly grated ginger
- Handful of Ice

Directions

1. Place the pineapple, orange and ginger in a glass

2. Mash barely to start to launch the taste

3. Pour the water over it

four. Let it sit down inside the fridge for two-four hours earlier than serving (or in a unmarried day for nice taste)

5. Serve in a tall glass

6. Enjoy your scrumptious wholesome drink

Peach & Peppermint Healing Water

Active Minerals: Potassium, Magnesium, Phosphorus, Calcium

Active Vitamins: A, B1 B2 B6 C E K

Other Facts: Contain fitness selling flavonoids and anti-oxidants. Mint is right for complications, nausea, digestion similarly to treating a number of exquisite ailments.

Good For: Healthy mucus membranes and pores and skin

Ingredients

- 1 cup peaches (glowing or frozen)
- 6-eight cups herbal spring water
- half of cup easy mint
- Handful of Ice

Directions

1. Place the peaches and mint in a pitcher

2. Mix together to infuse the flavors

3. Add water

4. Let it sit down in the refrigerator for 2-4 hours in advance than serving

five. Serve in tall glasses with Ice

6. Enjoy your scrumptious healthy drink

Lemony Lavender Life Saver

Active Minerals: Potassium, Magnesium, Phosphorus, Calcium

Active Vitamins: B1 B2 B6 Rich in Vitamin C, E

Other Facts: Lemons are correct for protecting your immune system. Lavender is outstanding for an disillusioned stomach

Good For: Good colon fitness and powerful anti-bacterial drink

Ingredients

- 6-8 cups herbal spring water
- 3 big lemons (lessen them into slices)
- 1/four cup sparkling lavender
- Handful of Ice

Directions

1. Place the lemons and lavender in a pitcher

2. Pour water over it

three. Let it take a seat within the refrigerator for 2-four hours earlier than serving

4. Serve in a tall glass with a sprig of glowing lavender

5. Enjoy your scrumptious wholesome drink

Strawberry Pineapple & Cinnamon Booster

Active Minerals: Potassium, Magnesium, Phosphorus, Calcium

Active Vitamins: B1 B2 B6 C E K

Other Facts: Low in energy

Good For: Anti-inflammatory and anti-growing old. The cinnamon is also exquisite for digestion

Ingredients

- 6-8 cups herbal spring water
- half of cup strawberries
- half cup pineapple
- 1 sage leaf
- Pinch of cinnamon

- Handful of Ice

Directions

1. Place the strawberries and pineapple in a glass

2. Crush the fruit slightly to release the flavor and infuse the water

three. Add sage leaf and weigh down a bit extra

4. Add water and cinnamon

five. Let it sit down inside the refrigerator for two-four hours in advance than serving

6. Enjoy your delicious wholesome drink served with ice

Watermelon & Rosemary Water

Active Minerals: Thiamine, Riboflavin, Potassium, Magnesium, Phosphorus, Calcium

Active Vitamins: B1 B2 B6 C E K

Other Facts: Watermelons lively in Lycopene which lets in to promote right pores and pores and pores and skin fitness. Rosemary particular for digestion.

Good For: Digestion, pores and pores and pores and skin, hydration & blood strain reduction

Ingredients

- 6-eight cups of natural spring water
- 3 slices of watermelon
- three sprigs of clean rosemary
- Handful of Ice

Directions

1. Place the watermelon and rosemary in a glass

2. Add water and ice

three. Let it take a seat in the refrigerator for two-4 hours in advance than serving

4. Enjoy your scrumptious healthy drink

Kiwi & Coconut Infused Water

Active Minerals: Potassium, Magnesium, Phosphorus, Calcium

Active Vitamins: A, E, K

Other Facts: Natural blood thinner. Coconut properly for weight loss

Good For: Anti-oxidant, bone strengthener, coping with blood pressure and boosts immunity.

Ingredients

- 6-8 cups herbal spring water

- four complete kiwi end result (peel and cut them into quarters)

- half of smooth coconut (which encompass juice)

- 1/four cup sparkling mint

- Handful of Ice

Directions

1. Place the kiwi, coconut and mint in a pitcher

2. Mix collectively to heighten the flavor

three. Pour water on top of all of it

four. Let it sit down inside the refrigerator for two-four hours in advance than serving

five. Enjoy your scrumptious healthy drink

Cherry Mint Health Booster

Active Minerals: Potassium, Magnesium, Phosphorus, Calcium

Active Vitamins: A B1 B2 B6 C E K

Other Facts: Anthocyanin's within the cherries act as anti-inflammatory dealers. Mint promotes digestion.

Good For: Inflammation, insomnia and complications

Ingredients

- 6 cups herbal spring water
- eight sparkling cherries (reduce them into halves)
- 1/four cup of easy mint
- Handful of Ice

Directions

1. Place the cherries in a tumbler

2. Rip the mint on the facet of your palms (this intensifies the taste) and upload to pitcher

3. Mix collectively and crush a bit extra

four. Add water and ice

five. Let it take a seat within the fridge for 2-four hours before serving

6. Enjoy your scrumptious infused water drink

Green Lemonade Tonic Water

Active Minerals: Potassium, Magnesium, Phosphorus, Calcium

Active Vitamins: B1 B2 B6 C E K

Other Facts: Green tea accurate for weight loss, diabetes & coping with ldl cholesterol

Good For: Detoxifying, energizing and cooling

Ingredients

- 6-eight cups natural spring water (warmth on variety until heat)
- four inexperienced tea teabags
- 2 lemons (reduce into slices)
- Handful of Ice

Directions

1. Place the inexperienced tea teabags in the warmness water and allow it steep for 15 mins

2. Remove the teabags and upload lemon slices (reserving 1 slice)

3. Let it take a seat down in the fridge for 2-4 hours earlier than serving

4. Serve in tall glass with sliced lemon on top

five. Enjoy your scrumptious healthful drink

Deep Berry Infused Water

Active Minerals: Potassium, Magnesium, Phosphorus, Calcium

Active Vitamins: B1 B2 B6 C E K

Other Facts: Contains Xylitol that is low in sugar and absorbs slowly in tool.

Good For: Weight loss, enables remove unfastened radicals and is also a first rate drink for diabetics

Ingredients

- 6-eight cups herbal spring or mineral water
- 1 cup of glowing raspberries
- 1 cup of sparkling blueberries
- Handful of Ice

Directions

1. Place the raspberries and blueberries in a pitcher

2. Mash the fruit slightly to launch the flavor

3. Pour the water over the fruit

four. Let it sit down down inside the refrigerator for two-four hours earlier than serving

five. Serve in tall glass with ice

6. Enjoy your scrumptious healthful drink

Cucumber & 3 Citrus Water

Active Minerals: Potassium, Calcium, Magnesium

Active Vitamins: A, B1, B6, C, D

Other Facts: Cucumber carries Silica which promotes bone health and the Citrus surrender result have excessive levels of nutrients C

Good For: Re-hydration, unique pores and pores and skin and hair, weight loss, digestion. Also stated to reduce horrible breath.

Ingredients

- 6-8 cups herbal spring water
- 1 big lemon (reduce into slices)
- 1 massive orange (reduce into slices)
- 1 big lime (lessen into slices)
- 1 cucumber (lessen into slices)
- Handful of ice

Directions

1. Place the 3 citrus cease result and cucumber in a glass

2. Mash barely to release the taste

three. Pour the water over the pinnacle

4. Let it take a seat down within the fridge for two-4 hours earlier than serving

5. Serve in a tall glass with ice

6. Enjoy your scrumptious healthy drink

Pineapple & Mint Refresher

Active Minerals: Potassium, Calcium, Magnesium

Active Vitamins: A, B1, B2, B6, C, E, K

Other Facts: Pineapples very rich in nutrition B

Good For: Indigestion and to boost immune machine

Ingredients

- 6-eight cups herbal spring or mineral water
- half pineapple (lessen it into wedges)
- 1/four cup sparkling mint leaves
- Handful of Ice

Directions

1. Place the pineapple and mint in a tumbler

2. Mash the fruit slightly to begin to launch the flavor

three. Pour the water over it

4. Let it sit down in the refrigerator for two-4 hours in advance than serving (or overnight for best flavor)

5. Serve in a tall glass with ice and a smooth mint leaf

6. Enjoy your delicious healthful drink

Raspberry & Lemon Infused Water

Active Minerals: Potassium, Calcium, Magnesium

Active Vitamins: A, B1, B2, B6, C, E, K

Other Facts: Natural preservative, aids in digestion

Good For: Great for keeping ordinary bowel moves and also unique for pores and pores and pores and skin and hair

Ingredients

- 6-8 cups natural spring or mineral water

- 1 cup easy raspberries

- 1 lemon (lessen into slices)

- Handful of Ice

Directions

1. Place the raspberries and lemon in a pitcher

2. Mash the fruit slightly to begin to release the taste

3. Pour the water over it

4. Let it take a seat down within the refrigerator for two-4 hours in advance than serving (or in a single day for splendid flavor)

5. Serve in a tall glass with ice

6. Enjoy your scrumptious healthful drink

Watermelon Cooler

Active Minerals: Potassium, Calcium, Magnesium

Active Vitamins: A, B1, B2, B6, C, E, K

Other Facts: Good supply of potassium that is an crucial problem of cellular and body fluids

Good For: Healthy heart and skin

Ingredients

- 6 cups water
- 2 slices of watermelon (reduce them into quarters)
- Handful of basil
- Handful of Ice

Directions

1. Place the watermelon and basil in a pitcher

2. Mash it up ever so slightly to release the taste and infuse the water

three. Add water and ice

4. Let it take a seat within the fridge for two-4 hours earlier than serving

5. Enjoy your scrumptious wholesome drink

Mango & Mint Infused Water

Active Minerals: Potassium, Calcium, Magnesium

Active Vitamins: A, B1, B2, B6, C, E, K

Other Facts: Mango rich in pre-biotic dietary fiber, minerals and anti-oxidant compounds. Mint is right for digestion and oral care.

Good For: Good digestion, hair, skin and beneficial aid to terrible breath

Ingredients

- 6-8 cups herbal spring or mineral water
- 3 big mangoes (reduce it into slices)
- half cup glowing mint leaves
- Handful of Ice

Directions

1. Place the mangoes and mint in a tumbler

2. Mash the fruit and mint barely to start to launch the taste

3. Pour the water over it

four. Let it take a seat down within the fridge for two-four hours in advance than serving (or in a single day for pleasant flavor)

5. Serve in a tall glass with ice and garnish with mint

6. Enjoy your delicious healthy drink

Melon & Strawberry Infused Water

Active Minerals: Potassium, Calcium, Magnesium

Active Vitamins: A, B1, B2, B6, C, E, K

Other Facts: Anti-oxidant and anti-inflammatory

Good For: Anti-growing old, perfect bone fitness and an extraordinary resource to weight loss

Ingredients

- 6-eight cups herbal spring or mineral water

- 1/4 cantaloupe melon (reduce it into wedges)

- 1 cup smooth strawberries

- four easy mint leaves

- Handful of Ice

Directions

1. Place the melon and strawberries in a tumbler

2. Add the mint and mash the fruit barely to start to launch the taste

three. Pour the water over it

four. Let it take a seat in the fridge for two-four hours earlier than serving (or overnight for exquisite flavor)

5. Serve in a tall glass with ice and mint leaf to garnish

6. Enjoy your scrumptious wholesome drink

Orange & Grapefruit Infused Water

Active Minerals: Potassium, Calcium, Magnesium

Active Vitamins: A, B1, B2, B6, C, E,

Other Facts: Grapefruit has large amounts of flavonoids and lycopene - all which help to fight maximum cancers and some of considered one of a type illnesses. Orange suitable for excessive blood strain, pores and pores and pores and skin and boosting immune machine.

Good For: Good normal drink for detox, bloating and digestive device.

Ingredients

- 6-8 cups herbal spring or mineral water
- 1 big orange (lessen it into wedges)
- 1/2 grapefruit (reduce into wedges)
- 1/4 cup sparkling mint leaves
- Handful of Ice

Directions

1. Place the orange, grapefruit and mint in a pitcher

2. Mash slightly to begin to release the taste

three. Pour the water over it

four. Let it sit down down inside the fridge for 2-4 hours earlier than serving (or in a single day for exceptional flavor)

5. Serve in a tall glass with ice with a single mint leaf as garnish

6. Enjoy your delicious healthful drink

Lemon, Strawberry & Basil Blast

Active Minerals: Potassium, Magnesium, Phosphorus, Calcium

Active Vitamins: B1 B2 B6 C E K

Other Facts: Anti-inflammatory and anti-ageing. The basil has excessive anti-bacterial houses

Good For: Good detox and useful useful resource to weight reduction

Ingredients

- 6-eight cups herbal spring or mineral water
- 1 big lemon (cut it into slices)
- 1 cup easy strawberries
- 1/4 cup of basil
- Handful of Ice

Directions

1. Place the strawberries and lemon in the bottom of the pitcher

2. Tear the basil and add it to the pitcher

3. Pour the water over it

4. Let it sit within the fridge for two-4 hours before serving (or in a single day for first-rate flavor)

5. Serve in a tall glass with ice

6. Enjoy your scrumptious healthy drink

Apple & Cinnamon Infused Water

Active Minerals: Potassium, Magnesium, Phosphorus, Calcium

Active Vitamins: A B1 B2 B6 C E K

Other Facts: Anti-inflammatory and anti-developing older. The cinnamon is likewise a excellent useful resource to digestion

Good For: Detox and actual for weight loss

Ingredients

- 6-8 cups natural spring or mineral water
- 3 easy apples (cored and sliced)
- 1 cinnamon stick
- Handful of Ice

Directions

1. Place the apples and cinnamon in a glass

2. Mash the fruit slightly to start to release the flavor

3. Pour the water over it

4. Let it take a seat in the refrigerator for 2-four hours earlier than serving (or in a unmarried day for top notch flavor)

5. Serve in a tall glass with ice

6. Enjoy your delicious healthy drink

Grape & Melon Infused Water

Active Minerals: Potassium, Magnesium, Phosphorus, Calcium

Active Vitamins: A B1 B2 B6 C E K

Other Facts: Grapes are a bladder cleaning fruit

Good For: Blood movement and constipation, stimulates metabolism and enables to burn fat

Ingredients

- 6-8 cups herbal spring or mineral water
- 1 half of cups grapes (reduce each grape in half)
- 1/four cantaloupe melon (lessen into slices)
- Handful of Ice

Directions

1. Place the grapes and melon in a pitcher

2. Mash the fruit slightly to begin to launch the flavor

three. Pour the water over it

4. Let it sit down in the refrigerator for two-four hours before serving (or in a single day for wonderful taste)

5. Serve in a tall glass with ice with a mint leaf to garnish

6. Enjoy your scrumptious wholesome drink

Raspberry, Peach & Kiwi Water

Active Minerals: Potassium, Magnesium, Phosphorus, Calcium

Active Vitamins: A, B1 B2 B6 C E K

Other Facts: Jam packed rich in vitamins and coffee calorie

Good For: Immune gadget booster

Ingredients

- 6-8 cups natural spring or mineral water
- 1/2 of cup easy peaches (use frozen if not available)
- 1/2 of of cup easy raspberries
- 1 kiwi fruit
- 1/four cup easy mint leaves
- Handful of Ice

Directions

1. Place the raspberry, peach and kiwi in a glass

2. Tear the mint and upload it to the pitcher

3. Mash the fruit barely to start to release the flavor

4. Pour the water over it

5. Let it sit in the fridge for two-4 hours before serving (or in a single day for first rate flavor)

6. Serve in a tall glass with ice

7. Enjoy your delicious healthy drink

Blackberry & Sage Infusion

Active Minerals: Potassium, Magnesium, Phosphorus, Calcium

Active Vitamins: A, B1 B2 B6 C E K

Other Facts: Sage recognised for its anti-fungal and anti-bacterial houses.

Good For: The darker the berry, the sweeter the juice and the higher it is in your number one health. This is that this form of outstanding juices that you can drink at any time.

Ingredients

- 6-eight cups herbal spring or mineral water
- 2 cups of smooth blackberries
- 1/4 cup sparkling sage leaves
- Handful of Ice

Directions

1. Place the blackberries in a glass

2. Rip the sage leaves together along with your fingers and add to the pitcher

3. Pour the water over it

4. Let it take a seat in the fridge for two-4 hours before serving (or overnight for awesome taste)

5. Serve in a tall glass with ice

6. Enjoy your scrumptious wholesome drink

Apple, Strawberry & Lemon Mint Water

Active Minerals: Potassium, Magnesium, Phosphorus, Calcium

Active Vitamins: A, B1 B2 B6 C D E K

Other Facts: Citrus stop end result are an terrific deliver of vitamins C and maximum of an apples nutrients are stored without a doubt below the pores and pores and skin. The mint within the recipe has authentic digestive properties.

Good For: Good for muscle swelling and stiffness and irritable belly

Ingredients

- 6-eight cups herbal spring or mineral water
- 2 apples (cored and sliced with pores and skin)
- 1 cup clean strawberries
- 1 lemon (reduce into slices)
- 1/four cup smooth mint leaves
- Handful of Ice

Directions

1. Place the apples and strawberries in a pitcher

2. Mash the fruit barely to begin to release the flavor

3. Add the mint and mash a touch more

4. Pour the water over it

five. Let it sit in the fridge for 2-four hours before serving (or overnight for remarkable flavor)

6. Serve in a tall glass with ice

7. Enjoy your delicious healthful drink

Mango & Strawberry Cooler

Active Minerals: Potassium, Magnesium, Phosphorus, Calcium

Active Vitamins: A, B1 B2 B6 C E K

Other Facts: Folates decided in strawberries assist enhance memory.

Good For: Good digestive health, detox and blood pressure regulator

Ingredients

- 6-eight cups natural spring or mineral water

- 1 cup of sparkling mango

- 1 cup of glowing strawberries

- 1/four cup clean mint leaves

- Handful of Ice

Directions

1. Place the mango, strawberries and mint in a glass

2. Mash the fruit slightly to start to launch the taste

three. Pour the water over it

4. Let it take a seat down inside the fridge for two-4 hours earlier than serving (or in a single day for first-class taste)

5. Serve in a tall glass with ice

6. Enjoy your delicious healthful drink

Orange & Mint Infused Water

Active Minerals: Potassium, Magnesium, Phosphorus, Calcium

Active Vitamins: A, B1 B2 B6 C E K

Other Facts: Orange is one of the maximum notably eaten end result on earth.

Good For: Good digestive fitness, detox and blood stress regulator. Mint extremely good for digestive issues.

Ingredients

- 6-8 cups herbal spring or mineral water
- 2 large oranges (reduce into slices
- half cup clean mint leaves
- Handful of Ice

Directions

1. Place the oranges and mint in a pitcher

2. Mash slightly to begin to release the flavor

three. Pour the water over it

four. Let it sit down inside the refrigerator for 2-four hours earlier than serving (or in a unmarried day for great taste)

5. Serve in a tall glass with ice

6. Enjoy your delicious healthful drink

Apple, Pineapple & Cucumber Infused Water

Active Minerals: Potassium, Magnesium, Phosphorus, Calcium

Active Vitamins: A, B1 B2 B3, B5, B6 C E K

Other Facts: Contains protein digesting enzymes

Good For: This very powerful water is a first rate for the digestive machine and furthermore re-hydrating the body.

Ingredients

- 6-8 cups herbal spring or mineral water
- 1/4 pineapple (reduce into slices)
- 3 huge apples (cored and cut it into slices)
- half cucumber (sliced)

- Small handful of sparkling mint leaves (non-compulsory)
- Handful of Ice

Directions

1. Place the apple, pineapple and cucumber in a glass

2. Mash the fruit barely to start to launch the flavor

three. Pour the water over it

four. Let it sit down in the fridge for two-four hours in advance than serving (or in a single day for excellent taste)

five. Serve in a tall glass with ice and mint to garnish (non-compulsory)

6. Enjoy your delicious healthful drink

Strawberry & Lemon Infused Water

Active Minerals: Potassium, Magnesium, Phosphorus, Calcium

Active Vitamins: A, B1 B2 B6 C E K

Other Facts: Folates decided in strawberries help decorate reminiscence.

Good For: Clean your tool and decorate immune tool

Ingredients

- 6-eight cups herbal spring or mineral water
- 1 cup of smooth strawberries
- 1 lemon (sliced)
- Small handful of mint
- Handful of Ice

Directions

1. Place the strawberries, lemon and mint in a pitcher

2. Mash the fruit barely to begin to launch the flavor

three. Pour the water over it

four. Let it sit down within the refrigerator for two-4 hours earlier than serving (or in a single day for remarkable taste)

5. Serve in a tall glass with ice

6. Enjoy your scrumptious wholesome drink

Raspberry & Lime Infused Water

Active Minerals: Potassium, Magnesium, Phosphorus, Calcium

Active Vitamins: A, B1 B2 B6 C E K

Other Facts: Lemons include limonene which has anti-maximum cancers homes

Good For: Good skin and internal health, constipation, cold and digestion

Ingredients

- 6-8 cups natural spring or mineral water
- 1 cup smooth raspberries
- 1 lime (reduce into slices)
- Handful of Ice

Directions

1. Place the raspberries and lime in a pitcher

2. Mash the fruit slightly to start to launch the flavor

3. Pour the water over it

4. Let it sit down within the refrigerator for two-4 hours in advance than serving (or in a single day for amazing taste)

five. Serve in a tall glass with ice

6. Enjoy your scrumptious wholesome drink

Iced Ginger Water

Active Minerals: Potassium, Magnesium, Phosphorus, Calcium

Active Vitamins: A, B1 B2 B6 C E K

Other Facts: Ginger has excessive anti inflammatory residences and is extremely good for the rest of joint pain

Good For: Good digestive health, gas and bloating

Ingredients

- 6-8 cups natural spring or mineral water
- half of cup smooth ginger (peeled and sliced)
- Handful of Ice

Directions

1. Place the ginger in a tumbler

2. Mash it up a chunk to start to release the taste

3. Pour the water over it

4. Let it sit down down inside the refrigerator for minimal of 3 hours earlier than serving (or in a unmarried day for excellent flavor)

5. Half fill a tumbler with ice and serve

6. Enjoy your scrumptious wholesome drink

Fennel & Lemon Flavored Water

www.ingramcontent.com/pod-product-compliance
Lightning Source LLC
Chambersburg PA
CBHW060500030426
42337CB00015B/1668